HEAD NURSE

HEAD NURSE

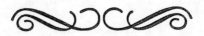

Barbara Villet

DOUBLEDAY & COMPANY, INC.
GARDEN CITY, NEW YORK
1975

Library of Congress Cataloging in Publication Data
Villet, Barbara.
    Head nurse.

    1. Nursing service administration. I. Title.
[DNLM: 1. Nursing, Supervisory. WY105 V748h]
RT89.V54   610.73
ISBN 0-385-02855-5

Library of Congress Catalog Card Number 73-22795

Though this book is essentially a work of nonfiction and the medical incidents it relates all happened, the central character, Margaret Striker, as well as the general medical unit of which she is portrayed as head nurse and the various staff and patients depicted therein do not exist in fact. They are a composite drawn from the author's experiences while working with a number of head nurses on units similar to 3H during the many months she spent researching this book in New York City hospitals such as Columbia-Presbyterian, Metropolitan, Mount Sinai, New York, and St. Vincent's, and where real people are portrayed their names and salient facts about them have been changed to protect their privacy.

For *Grey*

HEAD NURSE

Chapter 1

As the wheeled stretcher came careening down the hallway the IV bottles on the metal poles were clanking mournfully like bells on a horse-drawn junk wagon. The girl strapped to the litter was screaming and wrestling with the intern who trotted along next to her, trying to prevent her from dislodging the intravenous lines in her arms as the attendant maneuvered her past a series of wheelchairs in which elderly women, mildly surprised by the racket, sat tied in place for their afternoon "outings." The intern, Frank Richards, who had picked up his patient in the emergency room, was also shouting as several other doctors, including the floor's chief resident, Steve Newman, collected around him. Only the girl's husband was quiet. He trailed after the howling, clanking entourage, a look of stunned disbelief in his dark eyes as Margaret Striker, the new head nurse on 3H, moved to direct the stretcher into 319, a single room opposite the nursing station, which she reserved for critical cases.

It was three-thirty on a Friday afternoon in mid-August and though the new head nurse, who had assigned herself to evenings for a week, had just come on duty she was already briefed on the new arrival. Lucille Yaretsky, a twenty-nine-year-old mother of three, had been expected on 3H, a general medical unit in one of New York's largest hospitals, since about two o'clock. Sent in from New Jersey where an attending physician who had trained at this hospital had seen her, she was suffering from an unusual blood disorder called thrombotic thrombocytopenic purpura. In this disease the platelets, tiny guardians of the bloodstream that

1

participate in its clotting mechanism, are for no apparent reason triggered into a self-destructive chain reaction that cause them to precipitate minute clots throughout the body. Forming particularly in the brain and kidney, these tiny clots not only soon choke off the small blood vessels but also deplete the body's reserve of platelets so that in time hemorrhaging occurs unchecked, throughout the damaged tissues. When Lucille Yaretsky arrived on 3H the blue and purple bruises of superficial hemorrhaging that gave her lethal disease its designation, "purpura," had already begun to blossom on her arms and legs, and as the tiny clots formed and dissolved in the recesses of her brain her mind was guttering out.

"That poor kid," Margaret Striker said tonelessly to Stephanie Forester, the regular evening nurse with whom she would be sharing duty on 3H until eleven-thirty, when she returned to the nursing station. "I've never seen TTP before, only ITP; which looks about the same, but if the guys have got the right diagnosis—this version is almost always rapidly fatal." Her lips pursed in an expression of frustration as she glanced at the clock. "Look, Stephanie," she said, "you go on to report and tell Marie to begin without me. Newman or somebody is going to start yelling for help on the new admission in about two minutes so I'd better stay here for a bit. I'll get back to report as soon as I can. . . ."

Margaret Striker, the new head nurse on 3H, had been officially in charge of her forty-two-bed floor for only two weeks. Big and busy, 3H was one of four such general medical units in the twelve-hundred-bed hospital, rated among the nation's top ten, and only the acutely ill reached such a floor. Patients admitted here came through the emergency room, from the hospital's clinics, which ministered to the sick and dying of the ghettos, projects, and older middle-class neighborhoods of upper Manhattan, where the hospital was located, and by referral from outlying hospitals, for this was one of New York's great teaching institutions where super specialists practiced and their presence drew patients whose diseases, rare and common, could read like a list of the ways of dying.

Margaret Striker had originally taken over on 3H on a trial basis in mid-July, having been given the title of "acting" head nurse until it was decided whether she could manage an assignment considered to be one of the toughest in hospital nursing. On 3H, as on most such understaffed general medical units in major urban hospitals, the pace was grueling and the head nurse's position was pivotal in determining the quality of care patients received in a world of high-powered medicine that year by year was growing more impersonal and complex. A nurse with a cool, piercing glance that missed little and a reputation among her sister nurses for consistently superb performance, Margaret Striker, who had been promoted to her new job from a staff nursing assignment on a similar medical floor, had quickly established her skill and authority on the forty-two-bed unit and in August she had been officially put in charge on 3H.

The five interns, two assistant residents, and chief resident who were the doctors on 3H all were members of the hospital house staff, temporarily assigned to the unit as part of their training. In October most of them would be posted to other floors as the medical staff was shifted from service to service to give them a broader base of experience. But the nurses under Margaret Striker were the floor's regulars and, because she was the only person permanently in charge on 3H, the head nurse was expected to perform a staggering variety of roles. She was required to be a demi-doctor, equipped with a knowledge of the latest in medicine, drugs, and diagnostic procedures, a therapist and technologist competent with dozens of pieces of intricate equipment, an administrator, a records' keeper, a teacher to her staff and to the interns, a part-time dietician, a social worker, and, above all, a paragon among nurses, ever correct, merciful, and sensitive.

The doctors in this immense institution—as in most teaching hospitals like it—were being drawn further and further into the refined mechanics and abstractions of present-day medicine, so nursing had inherited many of the emotional responsibilities for patient care once exclusively within the physician's province. On 3H Margaret Striker had found that she often had to act as a

3

psychological anchor for both her patients and her own nursing staff in a sea of emotional turmoil. Every day on 3H held anguish of the kind Margaret Striker had just seen in Lucille Yaretsky's room and there was never any escape from the tensions that resulted among the unit's tight little society of professionals, each of whom coped with them in his or her own way.

Frank Richards, a voluble young man in any situation, emerged shouting from 319, loudly urgent about Lucille Yaretsky's need for immediate transfusions of blood and platelets to counter the insidious effects of her hemorrhaging. To assist him in getting blood samples to the lab quickly for analysis, Margaret Striker remained at the nursing station until the chore was finished. As a result she did not join the other nurses and aides from her day and evening staff who had gathered for report in the disused dialysis room at the end of their floor until Marie Velasquez, her assistant head nurse, who had run 3H that day, was well into her review of the patients on the A side of the unit.

"Jane is spilling three plus," Marie said, referring to the blood-sugar level of a diabetic who had suffered repeated small strokes since she had been admitted to 3H and had lain in coma for the past two weeks. "I've given her a tube feeding so you'll have time for Mrs. Teicher instead. She came off the respirator today and is afraid she'll choke to death if she tries to eat with the trach tube still in place, so stay with her if you can." She nodded to the head nurse but did not interrupt her monotone recital, flipping through the cardex file before her, in which each patient's medications and procedures were recorded, with a snapping motion of one hand as she rested her head wearily on the other. "It's wild in 322. Mr. Berman is out of his mind, as usual—they still don't know what's going on with him. Mr. Lee in B bed is clustering PVCs though Richards insists he's getting the dig-toxicity under control. He yells whenever you go in there to fiddle with the monitor. C bed is also a rule-out MI—Mr. Nelson—came in today with chest pain and he's still having it. No reading on his enzymes yet, Margaret." She gave the head nurse a meaningful nod before continuing. "James is going crackers in there listening to those monitors beep but so far that's his only excitement. They're moving him onto bleomycin as a poison tomorrow; the last marrow still showed blasts so keep your fingers crossed from here on cause they say this is *it*."

The litany continued, a recital of medical realities so understated and toneless that it was possible for the nurses, even as they mentally translated this verbal shorthand, to avoid its emotional impact. PVCs—premature ventricular contractions—the irregular heartbeats that can occur in the aftermath of heart attack and bring on cardiac arrest; MI—myocardial infarction—the result of blockage of the tiny coronary arteries that supply blood to the heart muscle which brings about its partial death and is known commonly as a heart attack; poisons, marrow—translated to mean a leukemic in a delicate and dangerous battle to gain remission from his disease by accepting the intentional poisoning of his bone marrow to kill off the cancerous blood cells manufactured there in hopes that normal blood cells will be produced to replace them. All these endgames with death seemed almost sterilized of emotional content by the medical language—though the head nurse accepted with an uneasy smile that Mr. James, a cellist, might well be uncomfortable as the audience for the dissonant chirping of monitors signaling the irregular heartbeats of his roommates.

At three-fifty, when report was complete, Margaret Striker and Marie Velasquez circled the ward on changeover rounds and though she stopped only briefly in each room the head nurse greeted each of the ward's patients cheerfully by name and her observant eye missed no detail in the appearances or surroundings of each that might provide a clue to his or her emotional and physical state. Jotting notes to herself on an omnipresent clipboard pad which she called her "paper brain," she seemed to fix in her mind every salient fact about each of her charges in a fraction of a second and file it away for reference as she went. But in Eleanor Teicher's room Margaret Striker tarried awhile.

A former chorus girl who had started in vaudeville at age eleven and danced for Ziegfeld, Eleanor Teicher was one of two patients

5

then on the ward suffering from a disease of the aged in which the bones can become so fragile that they can no longer support the body's weight. Some months before, she had coughed and her breast-bone shattered. For eleven weeks she had been partially dependent on a respirator to breathe for her while the lacy bones of her chest were encouraged to mend. Being independent of the machine today should have been a momentous occasion but, with a permanent entry cut into her windpipe to permit the life-supporting respirator to be hooked up immediately should another fit of coughing crumble her sternum a second time, Mrs. Teicher could not escape the frightening truth that in time, slowly, her legs would become too frail for her to walk and her backbone would begin to collapse downward upon itself. Yet with only the slightest encouragement Eleanor Teicher, for all her fears managed to be cheerful and her courage had won the head nurse's admiration.

"Eleanor," she said, squatting down beside the wheelchair in which the tiny woman sat, a look of strained worry in her expressive blue eyes, "you mustn't be afraid tonight. We'll stay with you every step of the way until you feel sure of yourself. You've been learning how to speak again—now you're going to learn how to eat with the trach tube in place, and soon you can go home."

Mrs. Teicher shook her head in a tiny, involuntary gesture of negation and began fumbling nervously with something in her lap. It was the framed photograph of a young man in a uniform recognizably that of World War II which she now offered word-lessly to the head nurse, a picture of her husband, dead for many years. Studying it, Margaret Striker's face softened in a look of understanding. Then, as she gently rearranged a wisp of gray hair that had gotten loose from the bright red ribbon restrain-ing Mrs. Teicher's curls, she said quietly, "He was a handsome man, Eleanor. And you must miss him still. Yet even when it makes us sad it's good to remember loving someone, isn't it?" Mrs. Teicher grew pensive and then nodded dreamily; she still had the look of a showgirl and her smile belonged to some-one twenty years old.

6

Moving down the hall, Margaret Striker passed the room with the one open bed in it that was left on the ward since Lucille Yaretsky's arrival—knowing that it would soon be filled. As she went she was quietly reviewing what she had learned on rounds, marshaling information on every patient and planning against each potential problem that might arise on the ward that evening. For with the sixth sense a good nurse develops, Margaret Striker felt trouble coming and though she did not know where it might strike, when evening and night staffs were spread so thinly— only two nurses and two aides on until midnight and one nurse and two aides to cover the ward thereafter—she made it a point to expect the unexpected. But her review of the forty-one patients on the floor did little to reassure her. Among those on the ward census whom she felt would require careful watching that night, in addition to Lucille Yaretsky, were two leukemics whose platelet counts were dropping into the dangerous ranges that might presage hemorrhage, one woman in progressive stroke, an alcoholic who might be bleeding internally, several terminal cancer patients, and a number of cardiac cases, four of whom were on monitors and six of whom should have been, had enough been available.

One of those who had had his monitor taken away that day was Mr. Desado, whose present stay on 3H had lasted several weeks. Many times a patient on this unit, Mr. Desado had suffered multiple coronary attacks which had so weakened his heart that his state was never "stable." On two prior occasions he had been resuscitated from cardiac arrest on 3H, his tired heart slammed from a standstill into beating again by a combination of pummeling, artificial adrenal stimulation, and electric shock, once after two minutes of "death." During his present stay his erratic heartbeat had finally been regulated by using a powerful drug called pronestyl. He had been in normal heart rhythm for three days and was scheduled to go home on the weekend if this was maintained—but, as Margaret Striker knew, anything could go wrong at any minute with Mr. Desado's heart.

When she reached Lucille Yaretsky's room the doctors were just completing their workup and it was perfectly clear from the

7

somber expression on chief resident Steve Newman's usually jolly face that the prognosis for this young woman was not good. As Margaret Striker entered the room, she looked up with the tear-stained face of a bewildered child and begged to be released from the heavy restraining straps that held her in bed to fetch her three-year-old daughter, whom she was convinced had been abandoned downstairs. Unable to distinguish between time and place, the young mother had no idea of where she was or why; her husband explained that evidently she believed she was at a hospital in New Jersey where a month earlier she had been admitted for an abortion and her little girl *had* inadvertently been left alone in the waiting room. This disorientation in time and place had begun to develop two weeks after the abortion, though within five days of her surgery there had been insidious signs that all was not well with Mrs. Yaretsky when she had begun to run a slight fever, complained of headaches, and at moments had been subject to a curious twitch that pulled her mouth askew. There was no hint of this distortion in the lovely Levantine face now—just a lostness—but the grim signs of her disease were visible in the huge purple blotches of superficial hemorrhaging that covered her legs, arms, and torso.

"We'll need constant monitoring on the blood pressure, Margaret," Steve Newman said to the head nurse, "and continuous use of plasma expander until we can get enough blood collected to send her for surgery."

"What is the platelet situation?" the head nurse asked, bending over Mrs. Yaretsky to fix a blood pressure cuff in place and beginning to pump it up while she waited for the answer.

"It's Friday," Newman replied tersely in what seemed to be a non sequitur, turning to leave the room.

The head nurse looked after him momentarily, her face suddenly as still as a stone in a reflex of self-control as she registered the chief resident's meaning. TTP, as Mrs. Yaretsky's terrible disease was referred to in medical jargon, had been shown to respond in rare instances to removal of the spleen, where, it was

8

theorized, the offending platelets were picking up their self-destructive instructions, coupled with huge transfusions. Mrs. Yaretsky was therefore on standby for emergency splenectomy but the surgery could not be performed without having on hand enough platelets to make up for her own depleted supply, and ten units of whole blood to replenish that which could be lost in surgery as well as that which had been steadily oozed away in the insidious hemorrhaging. And Lucille Yaretsky had picked a bad time to develop the full-blown symptoms of her terrible disease, for on Friday afternoon at four o'clock the hospital's blood bank would already be running short of certain types of whole blood and probably would be out of platelets. If that was so, Margaret Striker knew, Mrs. Yaretsky's slim chance at life could hang on a desperate shell game that was already being played all over New York City as hospitals began the weekend scramble for blood, trying to match supply at one institution with demand at another through the central bank. Some whole blood normally remained available in the commoner groups in the house store and frozen packed cells and plasma were usually in good supply until Sunday afternoon, but the rare blood types were often short on weekends and platelets with only a twenty-four-hour lifespan were almost invariably gone from the hospital's store by Friday evening. Obtaining them from the central blood bank took a minimum of three to five hours, and often much longer when a large supply was required after the commercial donor services had closed for the weekend.

In recent weeks there had been two deaths on 3H that had been at least partially attributable to the weekend blood and platelet shortages. A leukemic whose platelet count had been known to be dangerously depressed on Friday night had died of multiple internal "bleeds" on Saturday morning because no transfusions could be obtained for him for over four hours, and a "GI bleeder," as those with slowly hemorrhaging gastrointestinal ulcers were called, whose rare blood type had run out on Saturday had died on Sunday. If the hospital, working through the city blood bank, was unable to turn up sufficient platelets for Lucille Yaretsky in a few hours it seemed doubtful that she would live to reach the operating table.

Chapter 2

It was a difficult vigil for Margaret Striker in Lucille Yaretsky's room while the wait for platelets had to be endured. Patrolling 319 like a sentry, every half hour, the head nurse kept particular track of the young woman's blood pressure and urinary output. A sudden fall in her blood pressure could signal the onset of heavy internal bleeding while scantiness in urine production might mean that the kidneys, lacking sufficient blood supply, were failing in their function, a situation which the head nurse knew could produce lethal imbalances in Mrs. Yaretsky's blood chemistry that could kill her as quickly as a major hemorrhage. At five o'clock while Mrs. Yaretsky's husband was away from room 319, donating blood from which platelets could be spun down for his wife's surgery, Margaret Striker remained at the young woman's side, holding her hand and trying to reassure her that the child she feared was lost was indeed safe. When she was with her the pleading look never left Lucille Yaretsky's face—even as her mind seemed to slip further and further away and she began to talk to Margaret Striker as if the head nurse were her mother.

In the next hour time became arbitrary. It pushed Margaret Striker and Stephanie Forester through their evening routines at staccato pace. Medications were poured and distributed, meals passed, tube feedings given, temperatures and blood pressures taken, intravenous lines checked and restarted and new medications hung, diabetics tested for an overload of sugar spilling from the bloodstream into the urine, and Mrs. Teicher's first meal off the respirator was duly celebrated. Time moved in swift, commanding rhythms for the two nurses and their aides, drifted for those who lay imprisoned in their beds, and slipped onto a different plane for some like Mr. Berman, who wandered the halls wrapped in a blanket, shouting insanely. But time seemed to eddy with deadly slowness in room 319; as she tracked Lucille Yaretsky's slowly declining blood pressure curve into the third hour Margaret Striker registered her own increasing tension by developing a rash of hives at the base of her throat.

"It always happens when I reach stress-point one," she told Stephanie Forester as she left her at the nursing station to go in search of Frank Richards, the intern in charge of Mrs. Yaretsky's case. "By the time this night is over I won't be surprised if I've got hives from head to toe." A call had just come from the lab giving Mrs. Yaretsky's latest blood count; the report showed that her platelet level had dropped from the normal range of 150,000 to 450,000 per cubic millimeter to a drastically low count of 8,000.

The head nurse found Dr. Richards drinking coffee in the conference room with Eliot Cantor and Bill Fischer, the intern and assistant resident on call for the night who at six o'clock would take over responsibility for all the ward's patients from the rest of the medical staff.

"I'm afraid Mrs. Yaretsky's in big trouble, fellows," she said to all three. "She's down to eighty over sixty and, Frank, the lab has just given the CBC readings. They show the bottom dropping out on platelets. She's at eight thousand—and that was about an hour ago. If you're going to do anything—do it now. . . ."

Dr. Richards started to his feet, grabbed the conference room telephone, and set up an immediate appointment with the surgeons and hematologists—specialists in blood disorders—who were in charge of Mrs. Yaretsky's case. Shouting commands over his shoulder, he indicated to Margaret Striker, who followed him down the hall jotting notes, that he had only half finished his workup on a man named Gutzman, admitted that afternoon with a probable liver disorder.

"I'll see to Mr. Gutzman," Margaret Striker told him, "before I hand him on to Cantor. I just hope you get Mrs. Yaretsky to surgery soon or there'll be no point later on. . . ."

At seven-thirty a call came to Margaret Striker from the operating-room nurse. She was to prep Mrs. Yaretsky for the OR immediately despite the fact that the hospital's citywide search had obtained only two thirds of the full order of blood factors desirable for her surgery. After hearing intern Richards' report on the head nurse's meticulously charted record of her blood pressures and the latest lab readings, the surgical team had agreed to proceed with the splenectomy as Mrs. Yaretsky's only chance for survival—though the odds against her already were twenty to one.

As she lay sedated on a stretcher outside 319 waiting to be taken to the surgical building John Yaretsky bent over his young wife, oblivious to the swirl of visitors that filled the corridor. He kissed her hands, her face, her hair, murmuring to her words she could not hear. His young face was drawn with grief; he was trying to say goodbye. A priest was called and with a disposable pocket kit that contained holy water and oil he administered the sacrament of the sick. Then Lucille Yaretsky was wheeled off, the intravenous bottles that were still feeding Dextran into her veins clanking dully on their metal poles. John Yaretsky remained motionless and mute where the stretcher had been until Margaret Striker approached him. Silently taking his hand in hers, she led him to a lounge and after fetching him a cup of coffee from the staff kitchen she left him staring at an inappropriate quiz show on TV. As she left the room, a hint of tears was very close to the surface in her expression. Then, with a shrug, she shoved her hands into her uniform pockets and returned to the nursing station. There was nothing else the head nurse could offer John Yaretsky —no words to ease his fear or make his vigil less lonely, and because she knew how little hope there truly was for his young wife, Margaret Striker wanted to use her work to push away her own feelings of helplessness.

The head nurse on 3H was never idle for long. Not only did her routines provide her with a shield in moments when she felt herself peculiarly vulnerable to the anguish of someone like John Yaretsky, but she knew their usefulness. Like a sailor who diligently coils ropes, pumps bilges, and checks cotter pins in calm weather, Margaret Striker kept moving on the ward every minute, getting ahead of small, bothersome chores in an endless checklist which if left untended could, in times of crisis, create chaos. Part of her job was to anticipate and analyze the doctors' every medical need for their patients before they themselves recognized them, so that in stormy emergencies anything that might be called for medically was on hand and the unit would run smoothly no matter what contingency developed. "I'm a compulsive," she explained easily to Eliot Cantor, who began teasing her as she checked over the "crash cart" secondary drug lists in a spare moment. "It's not simply that I want to have everything under control around here because as a good feminist I intend to run my own show—it's that I'm frankly terrified when things start to fall apart. . . . I accept Murphy's Law," she continued, referring to a wry maxim usually posted in hospital labs for the edification of the technicians, doctors, and nurses. "I accept that if anything can go wrong, it will—and in the worst possible way."

At nine o'clock it was well that Margaret Striker's restlessness had put her ahead of the scut work of the evening shift, for when trouble came it came explosively and in several places at once. At eight-fifteen, just after visiting hours had ended, a new patient, named Herbert Bennett, had been sent up from the emergency room, accompanied by a set of X-ray films that showed that he had a viable lung space about an inch and a half in depth; the rest of both lungs was filled with fluid which registered as a white shadow on the plates. When Margaret Striker asked him when he had become short of breath the eighty-four-year-old Mr. Bennett admitted that he had had "some trouble getting around" for about three weeks but had been afraid to come to the hospital because, he said simply, "People die here."

A tiny black man with a grizzle of white hair, his face was that of a very intelligent gnome, an impression exaggerated by the oddity of his frail body set upon what appeared to be elephantine legs. In the month or more that Mr. Bennett's heart had been failing, fluids had pooled in his legs, blowing them up into huge trunks that pitted at Nurse Striker's touch. On first evidence, it was hard to understand why he was still alive, why his heart simply did not give up in exasperation as it labored against the growing congestion of his body and lungs.

"What's up, Margaret?" Eliot Cantor asked, striding into the room where the head nurse had lodged Mr. Bennett. "CHF?" The intern bent over the little man to listen to his heart and lungs with a stethoscope. "Rales," he declared, registering the crackling sound like someone crumbling cellophane which he heard as he moved the stethoscope to the base of Mr. Bennett's lungs. "Let's diurese him and put him on O_2."

"He might be a lunger, Eliot," the head nurse responded cautiously, "and if he's lasted three weeks this way I suspect he'll last until the blood gases come up on him. If he is a lunger, you know, you sure don't want to give him too much oxygen."

It was an easy exchange—typical of the relationship of this intern and the head nurse, for Eliot Cantor was one of the least aggressive doctors in the present complement, a young man aware of his own uncertainties medically and willing to listen to advice. It was anybody's guess—at the present moment—whether Mr. Bennett would be helped by oxygen or whether, if his lung condition were a chronic one, administering it might present a final blow to his tenuous defenses. Chronic lung conditions produce a curious reversal in the body's breathing mechanism, so that the patient becomes dependent on the poverty of oxygen circulating in his bloodstream for the stimulus to ventilate carbon dioxide from his system. Any sudden increase in oxygen can cause a "chronic lunger," as such patients are called in medicalese, simply to stop breathing.

"Okay, Margaret," said the intern, completing his examination, "we're between scylla and charybdis anyway so I'll compromise, let's give Mr. Bennett two liters of O_2 by nasal cannula, and start rotating tourniquets while we diurese him." To the old man, whose anxiety was increasing visibly by the moment and whose breath now came with a small bubbling sound, he added, "It's all right, Mr. Bennett, you're safe here." Then he pulled the covers

14

up around him, tucking him in much in the manner of a mother covering a sick child.

It was while Margaret Striker and Eliot Cantor were busy setting up to do an electrocardiograph on Mr. Bennet that buzzers began to sound insistently from the callbox at the nursing station. Checking on them, Margaret Striker found two lights showing on the intercom box, one on her side of the ward, from 324—a four-bed room where the delicate Mr. Desado was lodged, and the other on the opposite corridor, from the room that housed the leukemic Mr. Gaines, Mr. Berman, and two of the heart patients, Lee and Nelson, both of whose monitors had been recording dangerous patterns of premature ventricular contractions that afternoon.

Stephanie Forester reached the desk just as Margaret Striker opened connections to both rooms to hear a garble of shouts in which were discernible words like "collapse," "bleeding," "can't breathe," and "pain." In an instant the two nurses were running down the parallel corridors of 3H.

Stephanie Forester found Mr. Berman standing by his bedside urinating what appeared to be blood onto the white sheets. Margaret Striker, as she had expected, found Mr. Desado struggling to breathe, apparently in congestive heart failure. In the bed next to him, Mr. Gutzman also lay curled in a curve of pain, clutching his abdomen like a man trying to hold himself together. She swiftly sat Mr. Desado up, explaining to him in Spanish what he must do, letting his legs dangle over the edge of the bed to try to pool the fluids choking his system in the lower extremities, and pushed his tray table in front of him for an arm rest. Practiced with the procedure, Mr. Desado, his eyes as wide as fifty-cent pieces, his breath coming in rasping heaves, bent forward and rested himself as the nurse swung her attention to Mr. Gutzman. A rapid check of his blood pressure told her that it had dropped dramatically since she had recorded it at seven-thirty, but even as she lisened to the thump of his heartbeat with her stethoscope her practiced eye had read in his waxen face, wet with sweat, and the coldness of his touch the telltale signs of major internal hemorrhage.

15

"We'll help you," she said loudly and firmly, leaning to speak directly into the half-conscious man's ear. "I'm bringing the doctors *now*." She flicked a curtain around his bed to protect the anxious, inquiring eye of Mr. Desado from too much more excitement, then ran to fetch the doctors, and nearly collided with Stephanie Forester at the door of the room where Dr. Fischer had joined Dr. Cantor to finish Mr. Bennett's electrocardiograph.

Stephanie Forester's report indicated that Mr. Berman was in no immediate danger. His blood pressure was stable and, though he had evidently been slowly bleeding internally in quantities sufficient to have stained his urine with dissolved blood products, his situation was in no way comparable either to Mr. Desado's or to Mr. Gutzman's. Room 324, at the moment, was a crisis area. As the two doctors moved swiftly down the hall toward it Margaret Striker went purposefully into the medications room behind the nursing station and drew 120 milligrams of lasix into a syringe. "Get the crash cart down there, Stephanie," she instructed the other nurse, referring to the prestocked emergency unit used in cardiac arrest. "They can't give Desado 'dig'—so they'll diurese him and pray. But get Fischer to decide now if he'll call a code on him if things go sour."

She slapped the lasix into the staff nurse's hand and headed toward the supply closet to pick up administration sets and intravenous fluids—dextrose and water for Desado, a normal saline solution to pick up Mr. Gutzman's falling blood pressure. She knew that if Mr. Desado arrested or Mr. Gutzman was bleeding heavily enough to go into shock there would soon be need to call for an emergency team to help resuscitate the patient. The codes used to summon them through the hospital-wide public address system had to be called swiftly, for in situations of heart stoppage within three minutes cell death begins in the brain.

* * *

His knees drawn up against his belly, Mr. Gutzman lay shaking with fear and cold in his bed, barely conscious when the head nurse returned to the room. His complexion had already faded to the color of old snow. Bending over him while the doctors struggled to get IV implants in his veins, Margaret Striker listened for his apical pulse while she checked its rate against his radial pulse, taking the first reading over his heart with her stethoscope while her fingers measured the outward thrust of blood at his wrist.

"Pulse is getting thready," she reported in a quiet voice as she simultaneously fixed the blood pressure cuff in place, listening again for the rushing sound of his blood. "And he's down again, eighty over forty. . . ."

Dr. Fischer looked up, his boyish blue eyes wide. "Jesus," he said, nodding to indicate Mr. Gutzman's visibly swollen abdomen. "I'll get the type and cross-match sample, Margaret," he continued quietly, "and you call the bank and tell 'em it's coming stat."

Without a word the head nurse trotted from the room. "I'd guess aneurysm or the spleen," she explained briefly to Stephanie Forester as she brushed past her, giving two dreadful explanations for Mr. Gutzman's state, "and he needs blood just to *get* to surgery."

When an undiagnosed aneurysm—a ballooned portion of an artery wall which can develop under pressure—suddenly splits open the vessel lengthwise, blood is spilled into the body cavity as quickly as the heart can pump it out. The same is true when the spleen, without forewarning, ruptures itself and the portal vein that connects it to the liver and digestive organs. If either were the case, Mr. Gutzman would soon slide into irreversible shock as his circulation failed and heartbeat faltered unless both could be sustained until massive transfusions to replace the lost blood and surgery to staunch the bleeding were possible.

Grabbing Mr. Gutzman's chart from the rack, the head nurse opened it to the profile sheet filled out by Dr. Richards on admission through the clinic; simultaneously she dialed the hospital blood bank. "Sally?" she asked in a tight voice, still reading the chart. "Oh—she's off. This is Miss Striker—3H—clinical center—for Dr. Fischer. We've got an emergency. Gutzman's the name. Hemorrhage. We are sending a type and cross-match by emergency transport now . . . He's Mr. A. Gutzman, a patient ad-

17

mitted to 3H at three o'clock today. Please set ten units aside when you get the sample. Okay, I know the rules, but we've got a man up here who looks like he's bleeding out."

The first transfusion pack did not arrive on the floor for nearly half an hour. Mr. Gutzman, slipping toward death, was sustained meanwhile on intravenous saline solution. In the interim Dr. Fischer did an abdominal tap to determine what kind of fluid was pooling in his belly. As the needle punctured home, blood of a dark, venous color forcefully spurted upward into the syringe. Mr. Gutzman had either ruptured his spleen or infarcted it—breaching the portal vein—and without massive transfusions and surgery he would lapse into irreversible circulatory collapse within the hour. But when Dr. Fischer called for an emergency operation the surgeons were far from enthusiastic about Mr. Gutzman's chances, and an argument ensued between the medical and surgical service that continued through several phone calls.

In the interim Eliot Cantor and Margaret Striker kept working over the now unconscious Mr. Gutzman. Since the hospital ran by rules and the blood bank would release only one unit of blood at a time, the intern had run a marathon up and down the four double flights of stairs four times to fetch blood so that he and Margaret Striker could keep two transfusion lines running into their patient simultaneously. For a while there was a frenzied, electric tension in the room as the two young professionals struggled to hang on to their patient's life, but then slowly, almost imperceptibly, their activity began to wind down, as if a piece of film were being slowed toward the point where all motion must be stilled. As Mr. Gutzman's shallow, rapid breathing shifted into the long, lazy sighs that can signal respiratory failure the head nurse and the intern exchanged a bleak look that acknowledged that theirs had been an exercise in futility.

They sent Mr. Gutzman to the operating room anyway. Dr. Fischer finally prevailed on the surgeons by pointing out that with surgery Mr. Gutzman had one chance in ten to survive; without —none.

After he was bundled from the floor Margaret Striker stripped the blood-spattered bed, erasing every evidence of Mr. Gutzman's occupancy of room 324. She collected his possessions—a black suit, a shirt, tie, watch, shoes, underwear, striped socks, and a book entitled *Exiles*—and folded them neatly into a paper bag to be stored with one or two other such packages on a shelf in a locked closet above the desk where she did her records' keeping. It was a dismal little ritual and Margaret Striker went about it silently, then abruptly left the ward. She returned five minutes later, pushing a heart monitor before her.

"Where'd you get that?" Dr. Fischer asked, looking up from the desk where he'd been entering notes in patients' charts.

"Stole it," she answered, pushing it down the hallway. "It'll make Mr. Desado feel safer."

"Does it say Roosevelt Hospital on it?" Fischer inquired.

"Not this time," the head nurse responded over her shoulder as Dr. Fischer began to explain his remark to Eliot Cantor.

"We had a gypsy king in here one night with an MI and we didn't have a monitor available. That made the gypsies angry but after they'd shouted at us they finally got the idea that we weren't purposely neglecting their king but just plain didn't have enough monitors to go around. So they left. About an hour later, when the intern went in to check on the gypsy king, there was a great big monitor by his bed, a kind the intern had never seen before. It had a metal tag on it that said Roosevelt Hospital. The gypsies had just gone out and stolen it from Roosevelt and they got it in here without one person seeing it go by."

When Margaret Striker returned from setting up the "stolen" monitor for Mr. Desado she spoke of neither Mr. Gutzman nor Lucille Yaretsky. Instead, like a woman who straightens closets after some painful argument, she seemed purposely to engross herself in busy work as if to empty the evening's frenzied hours of their meaning. Only when she was leaving the hospital for the night did she betray any concern for either patient; she stopped to put a blanket over John Yaretsky, who lay sleeping on a couch in the lounge—still waiting for a word of his wife.

19

Chapter 3

Margaret Striker would try to forget Lucille Yaretsky and Mr. Gutzman over the weekend. Though as she left the hospital at midnight with Stephanie Forester she remarked that she was sorry she had not known Mr. Gutzman's first name so that in his last conscious moments she might have made him feel less like a stranger dying in the hands of strangers, she would not brood on this. Long ago as a student nurse Margaret Striker had recognized the need to build walls between herself and the dying—walls which she had never been willing to take down entirely, for she knew that her defenses permitted her to function in top gear medically, undistracted by anything but the immediate physical needs of her patients. This had not been a callous adjustment; originally it had been necessary to her survival as a nurse. But since becoming head nurse on 3H she had grown uncomfortably aware of how frequently the emotional needs of the floor's patients went unrecognized by the busy staff, and she did not yet know how to balance the compassion she often felt with the kind of clinical detachment required of her. For as a medical floor 3H was a place where few miracles were performed. Most of the patients who came to the unit could not be cured and medicine on 3H was largely a matter of adjustments—of extending life despite illness, of ameliorating pain, of coping with heart disease, leukemia and the many variations of cancer, and of helping those with chronic diseases to learn to live with their own limitations and those with fatal ones, to die. It was a wearing business, for every day she witnessed painful little dramas being played out like that which this past week had involved Mr. and Mrs. Lieberman.

An immense, froglike man whose pockmarked skin testified to adolescent unhappiness and whose lugubrious expression was, as it turned out, entirely justified, Mr. Lieberman had come in on

Monday for diagnosis of the cause of his "exhaustion" and gone home Thursday having learned that he had a terminal cancer.

He had been raised in Brooklyn, near the Navy Yards, in an orthodox Jewish family. He had married an orthodox wife who was homely, anxious, naive, and well-meaning. They had one daughter. She looked like her father.

All his adult life Mr. Lieberman had worked installing insulation at the Navy Yards. For the last two decades he had worked principally with asbestos. Now, at age fifty, he had saved money enough to think of moving to the suburbs of Long Island, where he had an offer to work part time with a commercial firm. He and his wife and daughter had been spending every weekend shopping for a little house with a big yard where they might "grow things," but recently Mr. Lieberman had begun to feel too weak for the Sunday visits to flag-festooned houses.

After several visits to doctors in Brooklyn he had been referred to the hospital clinic and from there to 3H. His X-rays showed a shadowy area throughout the lungs. It was known that many cases of mesothelioma—a cancer of the lining tissue of the lungs—had been found among the population around the Brooklyn Navy Yards; the cancer was attributed to billions of particles of asbestos insulation lodging like invisible threads of crystal in the lung walls. Mesothelioma was classified as an "industrial disease."

Mr. and Mrs. Lieberman suspected that he had cancer. He was, in his own words, "one of those people who never had any luck." He didn't complain; it was a bald statement of fact. But they did not speak of this to each other and neither ever used the word "cancer" with the doctors or nurses. Instead they asked in anxious whispers if it could be "serious," if it could be "cured," if there was "hope"—both knotting and unknotting their hands slowly, over and over in an identical gesture. But when Mrs. Lieberman was not at the hospital Mr. Lieberman would sometimes talk with the head nurse. Lying in the bed like some cursed prince charming, marooned in his frog form without hope of the princess's kiss, his eyes would fix on a place far from the sterile hospital environment and aloud he would wonder "if, perhaps, instead of a little house with a nice yard" he should spend his savings on a trip to Israel. "My wife has a sister there," he would say, his frog face dreaming. "She could remain when I am gone. My daughter too might have a place, a future, in Israel. . . ." But when his wife visited him they talked only of the house, the yard it would have, the roses she would grow.

His lung biopsy returned a reading of mesothelioma on Thursday—so advanced that the doctors speculated that his lung's interior wall was "like a sheet of crystal, white, sugary-looking, hopeless." . . . "I'd like to see it," said the surgeon, "just to see it, but there's nothing to do for the man."

The evening Mr. Lieberman left the ward his wife had walked in circles around and around the wheelchair as it was pushed down the corridor, her hands like a flight of birds as she celebrated her husband's "return to health." His daughter, following them, had been crying silently. It was a vision to forget. The wife danced, gesticulated, smiled. The daughter, well in the background, shuffled heavily, hopelessly, after them while around them other figures, like images from Goya's sketches, were crowded, staring without comprehending at their passage—the abandoned old people who seemed always to be waiting on 3H for visitors who did not come.

They were called "disposition cases," the sick elderly with no place to go. Brought to 3H from lonely walkup apartments in old neighborhoods where they had been left behind by now middle-aged children who seemed too often to live in some greenbelt suburb, there were always three or four such cases on the floor—cancer patients, cardiac cripples, victims of stroke, victims of time grown too weak to manage their own lives. They waited here, having won a standoff with some acute phase of their dying, for nursing homes to take them or to be sent to state-supported hospitals. Day after day they sat strapped in wheelchairs along the ward's corridors, some calling for help only God might give, some smiling at an inner vision burnt upon the mind long ago which now displaced the emptiness with pleasure, some still trying to cope with the present, reaching out with fumbling hands to stop the nurses as they passed and beg them to chat awhile. And one of these, Molly, had made Margaret Striker her friend by a magnificent ruse. The head nurse had become her sister-in-law, Stella, dead for forty-five years.

She must have looked like Stella; Molly told the head nurse that she did, and Margaret Striker knew it for the compliment it was, for when Molly talked of Stella she was transported back fifty years to a time when she and Stella had been young and beautiful, rich in husbands and children, living in the Bronx near a park well kept and secure even at night. Molly had filled Margaret Striker's mind with her memories of family scenes—of the children, round-faced and shining at tables heaped with holiday foods, of grand visits to hotels in Atlantic City, where they had walked the boardwalk in marvelous dresses of pale gray muslin and cream-colored silk. Molly had turned her into Stella. She questioned her closely about their mutual memories until the nurse had agreed to them, nodding, and seen Molly's blue eyes grow tearful behind smeared glasses so immensely magnifying that they pulled the blue forward into them like bowls set upon her parchment face, as she shook her head and wept. For she knew that Margaret was not Stella; knew Stella was long dead; knew too that she was dying now, piece by piece.

Molly was eighty. She had had a breast removed at sixty-five and with the strength that was in her had fought her way through three subsequent operations. She spoke of the struggle, of her horror of a radical mastectomy. She said it was like being half peeled. "Then the fuses started to blow," she said one day. "The superintendent couldn't fix them after that." Her arm ballooned into a grotesque thing and Molly, proud and still beautiful, had worked and worked to bring the swelling down, soaking the arm in a kitchen washtub with the water running over it while she exercised her hand with a ball. But during this time her husband's strength began to fade too. He was older than Molly, already in his eighties. She had dressed him every morning in a good suit and fresh tie, put a fresh handkerchief in his pocket and a fedora on his head, and set him in the sun in the park while she shopped and carried and cleaned before she retrieved him, for he knew he became lost easily and would sit and wait for her, afraid to move out of the sunny circle in which she left him. But later, forgetting even that he was to wait, he began wandering through the now unsafe neighborhood and Molly would command a troop of children—some of the tough new breed—to find him. When they did, she would go with them into alleyways and tenement halls to where her husband, Abraham, stood whimpering, for when he realized his lostness he would not move without Molly. And then Abraham died and Molly was left in the apartment with its jumble of photographs and books and dishes, and drawers into which she put, unopened, the boxes containing the new slips or sweaters or gloves sent seasonally by her children— one living in Chicago, the other in Washington—or by Stella's children, whom she had raised to see dispersed to California and Westchester. And slowly the cancer spread into her bones, checked only by radiotherapy which finally did its own damage, causing a breakdown of the brain's blood vessels and the stroke that brought Molly to 3H.

She was still in charge of her own life. She understood her pain —her tolerance of it, the length of time her pain killers kept her safe from it. She saved jello from meals to help her swallow her pills, hiding it in the bedside table away from the thoughtlessly neat hands of the aides who swept such prizes away. And then one day Molly had a second stroke and when she recovered consciousness she knew that she had been in a dark place, darker than sleep, darker than any memory of darkness, in which she could not see, hear, or feel anything. After that she became frightened of nighttime and cried like a child in her bed. Her cries, a mindless repetition of the stunned phrase "oh boy, oh boy, oh boy, oh boy," became so much a part of the reality of the ward that the staff seldom seemed to listen to them or to the weeping of others, whose calls, though different—one for her house, "My house, my house, want house," another for her children—were all the same protest against the night, a way to be sure one still lived, by hearing one's own voice.

In Margaret Striker's world these sad sounds went on ceaselessly beneath the general clatter and purposeful talk at the nursing station like some distant warning-bell tolling, and when they became unbearable the head nurse sometimes sought refuge by going to a window from which she could stare down at the people moving about in the project across the avenue, thinking how miraculous the children playing in the playground were, how superb the game of basketball, all curves, arching of the flesh, eye, fingertip interplay, mind in concert with body. It was the destruction of that kind of perfection that she dreaded when she heard Molly cry out; the singular miracle of life ended—movement, thought, dreaming, loving, being—stopped. It frightened and enraged her.

Long ago she had realized how incomplete every life must be —even at the very last—"That we live," as Wallace Stevens said in his final poem "in a constellation of patches and pitches-tinkerers without final thoughts, in always incipient cosmos." She knew herself to be made of unrelated chunks of experience—patches of life lived in a sequence that nevertheless did not fit together smoothly into a single unified whole. The child she had been, swinging on the dark branches of trees behind a white clapboard house, was partly lost to her. In her mind's circle she held intact only some of what she had known and felt and so too she had lost much of the girl who had come after the child. Lonely and shy, she was a dim stranger, someone who seemed perpetually to have stood just outside an enchanted circle where other children were happy. And what she had become was not so much the sum of these other selves as it was their new form—a young woman looking back to the child and then looking forward, but to what?

To finding herself one day as Abraham, whimpering in the hallways of a changed and frightening neighborhood? To accepting, as Molly did, fear of the dark?

She knew the fear had begun with the child. It was not a simple bedtime fear. It was one that recognized that a cold darkness persisted beyond the blue mantle of the sky's brightness. She had made the recognition on the edge of a frozen pond when she was about ten. She had been taken to a funeral that day. The school nurse had died. She had seen her body lying in the coffin and the terror she had felt had made her sick. Later that afternoon she had walked alone by a pond she frequented where ducks wintered. In the December cold some of them had been frozen into the ice and she had found them, some already feathered stones, some still struggling in a helpless frenzy to escape the stealthy cold that had seized them. In horror, she tried to free those ducks, creeping out in the profound cold of the early twilight to hack at the ice in such a state of rage that she had exhausted herself chopping dead birds from the black ice when no more could be found alive.

That same kind of rage had sometimes welled up in her during her first months as a nurse, echoing across the years, and she had felt then as the child had, the cold, the darkness behind the day's blue, the trapped helplessness of the old, the lonely, and the sick. It was this feeling, with her still though now quiescent, that sometimes led her to try to capture the unfinished past from the dying by imprinting their moments on her own memories so that they both might cheat the dark, stealthy cold that threatened all. And though with Molly this was sometimes accomplished—for there were moments when Margaret Striker could almost feel the lost breezes of Atlantic City fresh on her face and hear gray muslin rustling as Molly recalled moments when she and Stella had walked arm in arm along the boardwalk, young and heedless and happy—she knew it for the useless ritual it was, a remembrance of a crazy dance upon a frozen beach, and had resigned herself silently to what was happening to Molly, knowing that only by accepting it with her could she help Molly to find peace. And in the last weeks of her life—as if acknowledging that time was growing very, very short for her—Molly, through still terrified of the darkness, chose to muster her courage and take control of its ending in her own way. Each day, even as the perimeters of her existence closed in upon her, limiting her thoughts, her movements, her hours, she stood her ground by choosing to act as if that single day were the only day that had ever mattered to her. Whatever was still within her power to do, she did, simply, without asking to do more, and relinquished all else that was lost to her as if it had not been. Feeding herself, sitting up in a wheelchair, speaking coherently, keeping time in order—since these were what she still had the will to do, they became significant acts and Molly, deliberately performing each act, was heroic. But the day she was taken away to the nursing home where she would die ten days later she chided Margaret Striker and Eliot Cantor for having failed her in one way. "I wished," she said very slowly, staring up at them from the stretcher on which she was strapped in place, looking for all the world like a living mummy wrapped in gray blankets, her face utterly white, her eyes lapis lazuli, "that you could have fixed me up well enough so that just one more time before I see God I could have walked to the bathroom to wash my own face. . . ."

Chapter 4

When Margaret Striker took charge of 3H she had been a nurse for six years, long enough to lose most of her illusions about doctors, hospitals, and nursing, and to learn that what was wanted of her more than compassion professionally was self-discipline, stamina, and the ability to appear unruffled in any circumstance. Making her daily rounds, moving at the same clipped rhythms through days that ran into weeks on 3H, she went about her business in an obdurately colorless way, wasting no time on heroics or sentiment and expressing the compassion she felt for suffering primarily through her tireless efficiency.

But Margaret Striker had never lost the sense of how fragile life truly is, nor, despite her emotional restraint, was she as self-controlled as she appeared to be. She still grieved for the Mollys, she was often irritated when things went wrong on 3H, and she was passionately determined that on her unit the standards she set for patient care would not be compromised, for Margaret Striker had brought a strong will, as well as concern, with her to her assignment as head nurse.

Pale and rather lovely, with an early-American face wreathed in heavy dark hair like those often seen in oval-framed pictures of women whose grit had carried them in covered wagons across an unknown continent, Margaret Striker was a queer mixture of a girl—part flint, part tenderness. She had come into nursing not out of compassion for suffering but out of ambition.

The eldest of six children, she had grown up in one of those small communities in northern New York State that today seem to have halted time about thirty years ago and to exist there still —a town of white frame houses, maple trees, and neat lawns that speak of the innate sense of orderliness and conservatism of their inhabitants. Her father, a bookkeeper who, if his daughter was correct, had felt keenly the limits placed upon him by the lack of a college degree, was otherwise a practical, taciturn man who had demanded compliance from both his wife and his children. Her mother, who had remained at home while her two daughters and four sons were of school age, obedient both to her husband's wishes and to the conventions of the time, had nevertheless yearned for a different sort of life, and her undefined longing had filled the frequent silences that lay between her husband and herself. Margaret Striker could remember those silences—whole evenings in which neither parent spoke to the other. Her father would come into the kitchen on his return from work and sit wordlessly at the table while her mother prepared and served the meal and the quietness in the room became fearful. The tension of it drove the children into themselves—away from both parents— and because of it Margaret and one younger brother built a camaraderie from which they fashioned a private world neither parent could enter.

At first it was a child's world. Hiding in a copse of great evergreens that grew behind their house, sister and brother, riding the dark branches like horses, dreamed of going far away from the small town that was their home. But as they grew their dreams became more purposeful and practical, and though she appeared entirely obedient at home and at school, rebellion simmered in Margaret Striker's heart. For she did not let herself yearn for any of the things girls of her age were expected to want; instead of turning her thoughts in adolescence toward romance, she planned on a career in science or mathematics that would set her free of what she regarded as the entrapments of marriage.

A talented scholar, Margaret found a cool poetry in precise abstractions; form, order, arrangement—systems balancing systems— these were lovely in their own right and provided an escape from the disarray of adolescent longings that she felt could never be fulfilled in the strict, stern confines of her home. She excelled academically and her grades earned honors for her and confirmed her hopes of escaping to college. Assuming that she would win a scholarship, she never discussed her academic plans with either parent. But when the time came to begin applying to colleges and Margaret brought home catalogs from several institutions her mother told her curtly that there were no plans to send her away to school and no extra money to educate a girl even if she should win a scholarship.

Stunned and angry, Margaret, who had assumed that her parents recognized her ambition and academic talent as deserving of their support, began to look for a way out. Unable to realize that for her father the inability to finance four years of college for her might be one more admission of inadequacy and that in her disappointment he was reliving his own, she lashed out particularly at him and when she came to her decision to go into nursing she consulted with neither her father, nor her mother, for like most adolescents she was entirely absorbed by her own emotions.

Her last year in high school was a difficult one both for Margaret and for her parents. Often sullen and silent, she confided only in her brother and cataloged her resentments of her parents so that she would be well armed to make the break she felt essential to her survival emotionally. Her parents' protectiveness she construed as selfishness and their middle-class ambitions she disdained

29

as dull. Her father's symbolic securing of his home in hedges and fences and rows of trees Margaret chose to see as an attempt to imprison her, and she regarded his habitual silences as a deliberate refusal to communicate with his family. She did not realize, until she had applied to Johns Hopkins Nursing School in Baltimore and been accepted, that all the while her father had been carefully saving money to give her what he could to go away to school, and when she received a partial scholarship to Johns Hopkins he complimented it so much that, despite her mother's protests that Baltimore was too far away, Margaret was able to leave home at last.

Student nurses at Johns Hopkins, one of the oldest and finest medical centers in the country, trained for three years, spending their first year in classrooms and their last two years in rigorous training on the wards, where in twenty-four months they covered the major services of surgery and medicine and the specialties like psychology, neurology, obstetrics and gynecology, pediatrics, and orthopedics. Because the medical service at Hopkins had a reputation as the most difficult, Margaret Striker, characteristically, elected to begin her training there to prove to herself that she was equal to its challenge.

It was a fortunate choice, for until this time Margaret had regarded nursing only as a way to demonstrate her independence of home, and on the medical service she was forced to be involved with people as she had never been before. A scholar and a loner in high school, she had never made friends easily and never dated except for a single Sadie Hawkins dance, and though she had felt her isolation painfully she had taught herself to appear aloof and unconcerned. But on the medical service at Hopkins Margaret Striker found it impossible to keep her distance from people because the instructor, a woman she was to remember for years as the finest nurse she had ever seen in action, was a person of limitless compassion and sensitivity who insisted that her students become involved with the human as well as physical needs of their patients. Slowly, working with individuals, Margaret Striker began to push open a doorway to her own feelings that she had kept tightly closed since childhood, and years afterward she would recall her instructor at Johns Hopkins, Mary McCarr, as the woman who had taught her to listen to others for the first time.

She had been trying to teach a cardiac patient who was to be sent home how to take digoxin—an antiarrhythmic drug he would need to control the irritability of his damaged heart—but to her dismay the more carefully she instructed him the less he seemed to grasp what she was saying. It was as she initiated a third conversation with her patient on the subject of his medications that Miss McCarr called her from the room and began to question her about him. "How many visitors had he had that day," she had asked, "and who were they?" And what had they told her patient that could have upset him? To her astonishment, Margaret Striker realized that she had no idea how to answer Miss McCarr's questions and that she knew nothing about her patient but medical facts. Returning to the room, the young nurse sat down next to her patient's bed and asked him quietly if something other than his physical condition was worrying him. She learned that his mother—whom he had supported for years—was about to be evicted from her apartment because he could no longer pay her rent. She also found out that what she should have done for him as a nurse, before trying to teach him how to take digoxin, was to pay attention to him as a human being, for in treating him simply as a medical abstraction she had not only failed to earn his trust so that he would be willing to listen to her as a professional, but she had not seen the full implications of his disease in its effect on his life. Suddenly Margaret Striker had realized that a heart attack was not simply the occlusion of a tiny coronary artery that caused the death of a part of the heart muscle; it was a disordering of life, the destruction of a fragile system of emotional and familial checks and balances as well as of physical ones and she had realized not only how intricate is each human body, but how intricate also is the pattern of every life.

It was an insight that for the first time gave Margaret Striker some hint of what medical nursing could be all about, but with this sudden awareness of the preciousness of each life came a counter-reaction of horror with death. Though she had prepared herself for death as a textbook abstraction, she felt her defenses crumble when confronted with it as the extinction of a personality.

She knew why death was terrifying to her in these terms. The recollection still had the power to shake her years afterward and literally thousands of deaths later, when she had become head nurse on 3H. She had been nine—a chubby, lonely little girl who played clarinet in the school's junior band and admired the group's majorette, the daughter of the school nurse. The nurse, a woman of about her own mother's age, recognized Margaret's need for encouragement and treated her with warmth and kindness, inviting her for a visit, supporting her efforts to make friends with her own popular daughter.

She had seemed the perfect mother to Margaret, who had grown to love her. And then quite suddenly the school nurse was dead—of leukemia—in the space of a few weeks. At the time Margaret's own mother had been hospitalized with the birth of a younger sister. She had asked Margaret's father to take her to the funeral service for the school nurse. The coffin had been open and Margaret had seen her friend in it. She had bolted from the church and vomited.

As a student nurse Margaret had first tried to cope with the reality of death by refusing to think about it and so successful was she in repressing her fears that she was never afterward able to remember the first death she had witnessed. But she did remember the actions of the head nurse that evening. When the patient had expired the head nurse had come to Margaret and offered to help her wash the body. Margaret remembered that during the entire procedure she had watched the head nurse and never once looked at the body in the bed.

Caught between her growing sense of compassion and her own fear of death and dying, Margaret Striker learned to cope with her ambivalence by turning each death she witnessed into an object lesson in medicine. Training herself to think of why rather than who, she retreated, as have many doctors and nurses, into abstrac-

32

tions and began to see death as a challenge to medicine and to her own skills as a nurse. She could not yet afford to accept it as a natural counterbalance to life. Preoccupied with acquiring knowledge as a weapon against death, she became engrossed with the science of medicine and was, quite unconsciously, as fascinated as she was repelled by death as a medical phenomenon. And it was perhaps this half-realized absorption with the "enemy," as well as with the armamentarium of medicine, that led her, after graduation, to a post in a surgical intensive-care unit at one of New York's prestigious university hospitals.

Chapter 5

In every hospital the intensive care units are worlds unto themselves. This one—appended to a busy surgical service—was dominated by traumatics—victims of the city's violence brought back to life by surgeons' stitches after being gunned down, stabbed, hit by cars, or blasted by explosives. Margaret Striker, who worked nights, was expected to foresee and forestall crises like hemorrhage, shock, respiratory failure, and cardiac arrest, which easily followed on the double traumas of mayhem and surgery. There were only two nurses on at night, and with eighteen beds in the unit there were sometimes two cardiac arrests going on simultaneously so the young nurse simply had to perform. Using a medical approach to postsurgical problems, a kind of system-watch, she was so busy with all the "hardware" in the ICU that she seldom thought of her patients other than in mechanical terms.

Few patients stayed long in the unit and while there most were only half conscious. Drugged with pain killers, hooked to machines, tubes dangling from every orifice, they did not present a human aspect. The only time she remembered seeing anyone in the ICU who looked vaguely human was the night some gang members broke in to try to kill off one of the patients—the leader of another gang. They were driven out by the other night nurse, a black girl, who shouted them out of the unit in a language they understood, talking down their threat of guns.

Margaret Striker would later realize that she had been addicted to the fierce pace of the intensive care unit and hooked on crisis medicine in that year, but caught in a repetitive circle of routine, living by day in the provided nursing quarters and working by night, it never occurred to her that she was also slowly being desensitized by her experience. Instead, when she thought about it, she came to regard the ICU as a kind of testing ground of her skill and she was pleased to demonstrate her mastery of it.

One year later, having proven her ability to keep her emotions under tight control, Margaret Striker was invited to become one of six nurses in a new, experimental postsurgical unit being opened. Because nurses there were to be empowered to make certain decisions normally left only to doctors, she accepted the assignment proudly.

A tiny, four-bed section even further removed from the general hospital life than the ICU, the research unit had been set up to study the body's needs for particular proteins in various stages of trauma and recovery. To it—with their families permission—were consigned individuals so ravaged by violence, postsurgical complications, or combinations of disease and disaster that no more conventional treatment, either surgically or medically, was available to them. Offered a last hope in the form of experimental drugs and new approaches to regulating the protein chemistries of the body, they also received anticipatory nursing care that might counter death's delicate, early moves before they could develop into a final threat. In essence these otherwise hopeless patients were being used as test cases, for the unit was a frontier post in medicine where research and theory were experimentally applied to living patients, and when Margaret Striker went there it was still in its rough beginning phase—a raw, ugly place indeed.

Her first patient was a woman of forty-one, a Spanish-speaking mother of ten. She had been hit by a taxi, smashing bones here and there throughout her body and shattering her leg. The

34

doctors had fought for her surgically and medically but did not amputate the leg for fear that the shock of the operation might kill her. Finally, when the leg became gangrenous and abscessed, she was so debilitated by her long struggle that a conventional surgery to remove the leg in a fashion that would allow the stump to be closed would have been impossible for her to tolerate; they were forced to "guillotine" it, cutting it off swiftly and bluntly and cauterizing the raw stump.

In the unit Margaret Striker and her colleagues managed to keep their patient alive from September until December, for they swiftly learned how important it was to be aware of even the most minute change in the woman's condition and to make their decisions about treating her immediately instead of waiting for lab confirmation of a possible onset of sepsis. Abscessed from her leg to her diaphragm, she was continually threatened with rampant infection, and whenever Margaret Striker or one of the other nurses detected a drop in her blood pressure they would "plug in" the salt-poor albumen they were using as a plasma expander and begin to push antibiotics into her before her temperature began to rise. Anticipating the enemy before it appeared, they played their counterattacking game against death over and over for four months, until a fungal infection, resistant to all antibiotics, spread throughout the woman's body.

During this awful ordeal Margaret Striker had watched her patient's agony with increasing uncertainty and in December she began openly to question the ethics of keeping her alive. Finally she went to the resident of the unit and asked him why they were continuing to support the woman's life. The fungus had by then spread and sepsis was barely being held in check by amphiterycin and it now seemed to the nurse cruel to push the woman further.

"Why can't we just let her out of hell?" she asked the young doctor. "Why can't we just hold her hand and make her comfortable and let her go?" For the first time, though Margaret Striker knew that the purpose of the experimental unit was to find ways to prolong life, she felt that the doctors had gone too far in their pursuit of knowledge and she began to see how peaceful and merciful death might sometimes be.

Early in December she and another nurse approached the senior staff member in charge of the unit and told the doctor of their doubts. He agreed with them. A few nights later the woman's blood pressure began to drop. Margaret Striker, recognizing the signal of approaching sepsis, turned to the nurse on duty with her and asked her what she thought they should do. Both knew what the procedure would be if they called the resident: they would be told to put their patient on a plasma expander, push the amphiterycin, and hold on to her if they could. They decided not to call him. When they checked the woman an hour later her systolic blood pressure was sixty and they got no reading on the diastolic; she had slipped from a semi-conscious drugged agony into a coma. Her face then was more peaceful than Margaret Striker had ever seen it.

Of the 150 cases Margaret Striker nursed on the unit more than 100 died and though most of them were simply taken swiftly and irrevocably, there were enough whose agony was prolonged to leave the awesome question of where medicine should stop and the rights of the dying be considered unanswered in Margaret Striker's mind, especially after she saw one of her patients live through hell and recover.

A fifty-year-old grandfather whose daughter-in-law had been killed in an automobile accident had been helping his son raise his six children until he too was struck down by a car. When brought to the experimental unit the man was past "hope," massively abscessed. As his long ordeal continued it seemed to Margaret Striker that once again she was a party to a doubtful experiment with human life much like that which had caused the long, blind agony of her first patient. But when she again questioned the right of the doctors to continue treating this man she was told that since every experimental possibility had not yet been exhausted the doctors were morally bound to proceed. In the end, when he walked away from the hospital, the young nurse discovered that she had no answers for her own dilemma on the unit except that she knew she must leave it. She had kept herself going through months of apalling service by telling herself that she was contributing to a work directed at developing new drugs which saved lives, and in time she did see many of the experimentals tried out there, like carbonicillin and gentomycin, in general use. But she had also let herself be driven day after day by the sheer challenge of the work and had done many things without questioning them. And as she began to wonder about who lived and who died, about what it meant to be a patient, Margaret Striker realized that she had somehow lost her way as a nurse in the last two years.

Chapter 6

In the haunting April morning, walking home from the hospital as spring sketched its tentative promises in the pale fountains of forsythia, Margaret Striker began to realize how narrowly circumscribed her life had become. Swallowed in routine, she was no more than a cipher in an immense hospital, isolated and troubled with the grim work she did each night. Though she had cultivated a kind of numbness while at work she was finding that awful visions sometimes rose in her head when she was not on guard and she surprised herself one morning—when she thought herself as empty of feelings as a machine—by beginning to cry. Later, after she had spent some time trying to analyze why, she realized that she was enraged by what had been happening to her, and that by responding to every challenge that had been put before her as a nurse, she had let herself be used by a system that seemed to depend precisely on this kind of professional response from nurses to get its toughest work done.

Though she did not then realize it, Margaret Striker's reactions repeated a familiar pattern in the nursing profession. A gifted practitioner, she had been thrust into the hardest jobs because she was competent and with true professional pride she had proven herself equal to the worst demands. Now, her sensibilities exhausted, her emotions in turmoil, she had reached a state in which she needed a change as much to refresh her spirit as to overcome her resentment. That spring, when she began to look for a new job, she intended to use her diploma as a pass to help her find a new life in a new city as much as a new challenge in nursing.

Drawn first to San Francisco and Denver, she began job hunting by visiting their major medical centers, only to discover that, contrary to most cities, these two because of their physical and cultural attractions enjoyed an overabundance of RNs, most of whom held bachelor's degrees. The experience brought Margaret Striker to the disappointing realization that her own three-year diploma from Johns Hopkins lacked the "status" of a baccalaureate degree and that for all her specialized experience in intensive care, she might need to upgrade her degree if she was to compete for advancement in nursing.

It was the spring of 1969. That year the race for credentials in nursing had been intensified by an experiment aimed at stabilizing the nursing staff in any given hospital by changing the licensing procedures; it was being tried in Chicago. Designed in part to retain nurses in the hospitals from which they graduated, the move, supported by the powerful forces of HEW, the Hospital Administrators Association, and the AMA, was designed to give these institutions per se, instead of state boards of examiners, the right to license nurses. Opposed by most nursing organizations because it would take freedom of movement away from the profession, the threat made it clear that to hold on to their right to statewide licensing and reciprocity similar to those conferred on doctors and lawyers, nursing would have to upgrade its credentials to protect itself.

It was for these reasons that, in 1969, any ambitious nurse who looked to the future realized that leadership roles in her profession would soon be restricted to those holding advanced degrees—the more the better, and this new fact of life had a direct bearing on Margaret Striker, who now realized that no matter how well qualified she might be personally, she could not compete for pay

38

or position in the hierarchy of nursing without further education. Much as her father had been, she would be automatically classified as less intelligent and less competent because she lacked on-paper proof of her talents. The realization added a new dimension to her job search, and in the end it was the rich university life of Boston that influenced her to take a job there.

The following autumn she signed on for night duty at one of Boston's most prestigious hospitals. The job seemed to suit her needs perfectly. It combined freedom to pursue studies by day with a new challenge in nursing, for attached to the seventeen-bed medical intensive-care section to which she was assigned was a four-bed coronary care unit and as part of her assignment she was offered the chance to train as a CCU nurse, in anticipation of becoming one of the staff in a new eight-bed coronary care unit opening in a few months.

In 1969, coronary care units were becoming standard equipment in large hospitals across the nation. Developed in response to the fact that of the 500,000 deaths annually due to heart attack in the United States, half were unnecessary and resulted from sequels to the primary attack signaled by erratic heartbeats, called arrhythmias, or other recognizable symptoms, the units were staffed and equipped to identify and treat such emergencies as they developed. Monitoring the machines that monitored their patients, the coronary care nurses were legally empowered to make medical decisions and to act upon them in the absence of doctors, and though they followed the treatment programs prescribed in each situation, they could and did decide on their own when to act in each of the heart's crises, which drugs to use, and when to administer precordial electric shock through the chest wall to convert threatening rhythms to safe ones. In recognition of their special skills, CCU nurses were regarded as an elite in their own profession and accorded a respect by doctors few nurses enjoyed.

It was as much a hunger for recognition as the challenge of this advanced nursing that drew Margaret Striker to train for coronary care, but almost as soon as she had begun to work on the

39

huge intensive care unit she realized that she was once more taxing herself beyond her strength. By itself the work in the intensive care section used up most of her energies; with seventeen crisis patients in the unit and four more in the coronary care section, Margaret Striker found herself on the run most of the night simply to get her basic work done. Just as it had been in New York, the ICU was a place of frenzied activities; often several cardiac arrests were going on simultaneously in both the ICU and the CCU, so the four nurses and four interns on night duty seldom had time to sit down. To control their own tensions the young doctors and nurses sometimes played volleyball in the unit hallway just to rid themselves of nervous highs, and at this pace it did not take Margaret Striker long to realize that she could not carry a full load of outside academic work, train for CCU, and do her job decently in the ICU as well. Predictably, she dropped her studies.

Having given up her pursuit of degree, Margaret Striker concentrated on preparing herself for coronary care as a nursing specialty—but when the new unit opened in January she still did not feel she had either the skill or the experience she needed to work there. She found it quite a different thing to *know* theory than to *practice* it; though she could read normal sinus rhythm on the cardiac monitor scopes when she went up to the CCU and was able to recognize "bad" rhythms when she saw them on a ECG strip, she did not have the kind of knowledge she needed to feel secure.

On her second night in the new coronary care unit, at three o'clock in the morning, dangerous episodes of rapid beating appeared on the heart monitoring scope of a bus driver who had suffered a heart attack just after arriving in Boston, from New York, earlier that evening. Acting swiftly, Margaret Striker drew lidocaine, an antiarrhythmic drug, into a syringe for a push intravenous injection and then measured a second amount into a mixture of dextrose and water for a slow intravenous drip infusion —all the time staring fixedly at the scope in front of her, which showed that her patient's erratic episodes of rapid heart rhythm were coming in close salvos. She had been told the location of the damage to his heart and knew that it was dangerous. The blood supply had been cut off to the posterior wall of the left ventricle—the portion of the heart that pumps freshened blood to the body and back to the heart muscle itself via the coronary arteries that arise from the aorta—and he was vulnerable to rapidly developing ventricular tachycardia—a very fast beating of the ventricles which can easily wear out the heart or precipitate cardiac arrest. After she had given him the lidocaine she stood staring fixedly at the screen, watching the heart rhythm traced there by a bouncing light that traveled along an erratic pathway.

As the tachycardia abated she realized that she was terrified; she was unable to swallow, felt icy-cold, and her hands were shaking badly. There was another CCU nurse on duty with her, but somehow Margaret Striker could not turn to her and say, "I'm scared." Instead, she reached for the phone and began dialing the number of the intern on call—Jeff Washington. He answered and she said, "Jeff, I'm frightened. Sleep in the unit tonight." He came five minutes later with a mug of coffee for her and found her still hypnotized by the screen, afraid to see anything there that might signal the beginning of the end for the bus driver.

Jeff Washington, tall, slim, and toothy and one of the two black interns in training at the hospital, was a young man so delighted with life that he was given to impromptu recitations of his own poetry as he made rounds. Margaret Striker had worked with him in intensive care, and though they were temperamentally very different she liked him both as a doctor and as a person. When he arrived in the CCU, giving her a friendly hug when he saw the look of anxiety on her face, she felt both relieved and delighted.

The bus driver survived the night, though not without several recurrences of potentially dangerous arrhythmias that kept the intern and nurse watching his monitor scope till dawn. During the long vigil, despite her tension, Margaret Striker found herself talking with Jeff Washington as she had seldom talked with any other young man except her own brother. As she told him of

41

the last grim year in New York she heard herself saying things she had never allowed herself to express—about her loneliness, about her feelings of insecurity both as a nurse and a young woman, about her struggles to prove herself through her work and her doubts about her competence for her present assignment. He had listened with sympathy, pushing her quietly to talk out her feelings, insisting that she should take pride both in her skill as a nurse and in herself as a woman. "You're a pretty girl, Margaret," he told her, "and a smart one too. Ain't nothing wrong with you, baby." It was the first time anybody had ever told her she was pretty.

The strange intimacy of the unit by night drew them together. The quietness ticked with the erratic rhythms of sick hearts and the scrawling lights on the scopes spelled out messages of life's brevity and the folly of wasting it. It was an atmosphere that enhanced a mutual awareness between the intern and the nurse and made it possible for them to regard each other simply as friends—young people who had much in common.

Chapter 7

It was on a Sunday in March, when Margaret Striker was working evenings and Jeff Washington, who had signed up for an extra month of concentration in cardiology as an elective and was attached to the unit, was also on duty, that a call came to CCU that Margaret Striker was later to remember with amazing clarity, not only because of the fanfare that surrounded the admission of John Bartlett to the specialized coronary care section but because his arrival there opened a new chapter in her life.

CCU had been full that evening but before the resident physician who was admitting put the phone down he had decided to make room for John Bartlett. The fifty-year-old industrialist was in the last phases of what seemed to be a massive heart attack which almost certainly would be followed by potentially killing arrhythmias. Without the special kind of care only a coronary unit could provide Bartlett's chances for survival would be cut by half. Realizing this, the resident had decided to push a woman who had been scheduled for discharge to a ward bed the next day out of CCU twelve hours earlier than had been planned.

The transfer required that a mechanical pacemaker, set into the woman's heart some five days earlier by running a line through the superior vena-cava—the large vein that carries blood back to the heart's right side, where signals controlling a normal heartbeat originate—be removed. The pacemaker was a temporary implant, "on call" to deliver corrective jolts of electricity to the patient's heart only when its natural pacing became erratic. It had not been triggered for several days; the woman had been in normal sinus rhythm for sixty-eight hours, so her healthy heartbeat seemed well established. There was therefore no reason to anticipate any trouble as a result of pulling the pacemaker twelve hours early. As the cardiology resident, Jeff Washington, and Margaret Striker began the delicate job of withdrawing it they were unconcerned. But as the resident began to manipulate the line in preparation for slowly pulling the miniature electrode mounted on a catheter tip out of the heart's right atrium and up through the vein to exit in the arm Margaret Striker noticed something peculiar in the tracings on the woman's electrocardiograph, which was being run as a precautionary measure. The pacemaker's signal had begun to look queer and when she called this to the resident's attention the young doctor stared at it to realize, with horror, that somehow the catheter had punctured the heart wall. The signal—a tiny electric blip—was coming from outside the heart, from the interspace between it and the pericardium— the protective sac that gloves the heart so that it floats in a thin layer of serum.

There was a quiet pause as the three looked at the signal and one another. Unsure of *what* had happened, Margaret Striker knew that something was wrong. Then as the resident began to withdraw the line and she and Jeff watched the ECG printout, it was all there. The pacemaker signal emerging through the heart wall, back into the right atrium, and up and out of the heart—a perfect record of heart puncture in reverse. Had the woman's infarction been on the right side—had the pacemaker gone through "dead" tissue—the heart could have ruptured then and there. But as it was the pacemaker had gone out and been pulled back through healthy tissue, like a needle going through a piece of elastic. The heart gave a few complaining shouts of arrhythmia, the woman thought she was having another heart attack, and it was over. The only real protest the three heard about the whole thing came a little later from the resident out on the ward waiting to receive the transfer. He complained that it was a little late to be sent a lady with a left ventricular MI, a newly acquired, right-sided heart puncture, and "the psychotic attitude that something was wrong with her," and Margaret Striker herself thought that the woman had been treated rather badly until she saw Bartlett. There wasn't any question in her mind then that the resident had done the right thing in transferring the woman. Bartlett was in desperate need and no one in the coronary care unit that evening knew why he had not already expired.

John Bartlett was in visible pain as he was wheeled into the unit on a stretcher, his face ashen and filmed with a cold sweat. Margaret Striker, receiving him, instantly gave him oxygen, set up the electrocardiograph machine built into the wall unit at his bedside and began running a twelve-section tracing on his heart that told her at a glance that Bartlett had probably done considerable irreversible damage to his heart and was going to need constant surveillance in the next few critical hours.

She knew that not even a cardiologist was ever sure about a myocardial infarction from an electrocardiograph alone. To determine the full extent of the damage to Bartlett's heart the doctors would need solid readings on enzymes the dying cardiac tissue produces for several days after an infarction, matched with serial electrocardiographs taken during the same period. But Bartlett's story was the kind that left the nurse with little doubt that he'd had a massive myocardial infarction.

Handsome and keenly intelligent, John Bartlett was in many

ways a classic study of the All-American Heart Attack. Though he held a medical degree he had never practiced medicine, but had made himself wealthy in an allied field by driving himself hard. A self-made man, he prized his success and had enjoyed its rewards lavishly in the form of a high style of living, a jet-age schedule of work and play, an impending divorce, and a beautiful mistress whom he intended to marry. The only things missing in a curriculum vitae that spelled "coronary" were that Bartlett was neither hypertensive nor did he smoke. He appeared fit, looked younger than his fifty years, and seemed to deny any threat to his well-being. Even after experiencing crushing pain in his chest for several hours he was still alert and almost charming on his arrival in the unit, and had asked Margaret Striker about the seriousness of his state in the gentle yet undeniably forceful voice of a man used to getting favorable answers to any questions he asked.

But Bartlett had already had several warnings that all was not well with his heart—warnings he had chosen to dismiss even as recently as the previous Friday night, when he had experienced a heavy pain in his chest while flying from Chicago to Boston. Diagnosing it as tension indigestion, he had treated himself with a stiff three fingers of bourbon on reaching his apartment and the pain had subsided, leaving only a restless anxiety in its wake that had kept Bartlett sleepless much of the night. Irritable the next morning, he had quarreled with his lady friend and she had stalked angrily out of the suite he kept for them in Boston.

That afternoon, when the pain had repeated and become more fierce, Bartlett had called a cardiologist and gone to his office. He was told then that his electrocardiograph indicated that he had probably suffered an occult myocardial infarction some months before and that his present discomfort could be the danger signals of more trouble impending. The cardiologist wanted to hospitalize him immediately but Bartlett had refused and gone back to his apartment.

That Saturday evening, when the pain had begun again, Bartlett who had been given prescriptions of seconal and demerol, had taken both—and then walked the floor until the combined sedative and pain killer had let him sleep. But by Sunday afternoon he could no longer deny that he was having a heart attack. The pain in his chest had become a crushing, squeezing horror that radiated upward into his jaw and left shoulder, then down his arm, leaving him wet with sweat and sick to death. He had called the cardiologist, who had arranged for an ambulance; the attendants were just carrying him from the apartment when his girl friend returned.

John Bartlett's reactions to his heart attack had been classic; many of those who die of coronary occlusions do so because they refuse to accept the seriousness of their own pain and fail to call for help in time. Even after they are brought to hospitals, close to half of the patients who find themselves in coronary care unit, will deny that they have sustained any damage to their hearts. Some reject their mortality so powerfully that when they leave the unit they have no recollection of ever having been there or of their heart attacks. In Margaret Striker's experience, patients whom she nursed could not recall her face when she went to visit them in the weeks of recuperation in the hospital after their stay in CCU. Others were angry with what had happened to them, rejecting the insult to their hearts by rejecting the professionals and hospital that tried to help them. But denial and anger were useless defenses for John Bartlett; the messages were written there, scrawled across his monitor scopes. And Bartlett —despite his first wish to reject what had happened—knew very soon after his arrival that death might be very near.

Working with him in those first hours in the unit, Margaret Striker began to realize that beneath his calm, urbane surface John Bartlett was afraid and casting about for psychic lifelines. Deliberately the young nurse had begun to supply them. Like actors in some stylized play, they had woven together the roles of nurse and patient as if the pattern of the relationship were preordained, building an invisible series of connections between themselves that allowed John Bartlett to slowly relinquish his independence and accept that in the next six hours, when he would be most vulnerable to killing arrhythmias, this cool but caring girl would be the guardian of everything he knew and loved.

That evening, watching Bartlett and his girl friend, who was half kneeling by his bed on a low stool, holding his hand, her head resting against his leg, a look of intolerable sadness on her face, Margaret Striker felt her heart go out to both of them. For in the woman's face she saw the vulnerability of love and though she wanted to help she knew there was nothing she could do but stand there watching Bartlett's monitor, making herself familiar with the beat so that she would recognize the slightest change in its pattern while she waited for the hundred milligrams of demerol she had given him to knock him out.

Near eleven that night, after the resident had persuaded John Bartlett's friend to go home and had himself left the hospital, Bartlett's monitor began to register ugly clusters of premature ventricular contractions. The ECG had located the newly damaged portion of the heart muscle on the anterior wall of the left ventricle—the chamber that pumps freshened blood to the body—and with it shown signs of earlier slighter heart damage on the opposite wall. Paired with the present muscle destruction, the infarctions had resulted in partial blockage of the signals which synchronize the heart's beat—a dangerous situation that almost guaranteed that Bartlett's heart function would become increasingly erratic.

On duty with two other nurses, Margaret Striker felt a prickle of anxiety when she looked at the new rhythm strips taken on Bartlett; they recorded several extended intervals of premature ventricular contractions. She drew lidocaine for an immediate infusion, set up a second dose of this antiarrhythmic drug for prolonged drip intravenously, and dialed Jeff Washington, who was on duty, to warn him that trouble seemed to be on the way. As she put the phone down she glanced toward Bartlett's cubicle; he was staring straight into her eyes. The look seemed to probe her and she felt her own heart leap involuntarily as his expression changed suddenly from a look of intentness to one of frozen amazement and his heart monitor began to bell a repeated danger call.

When Jeff Washington arrived on the unit minutes later, Margaret Striker and another CCU nurse had already made the first emergency moves to prevent Bartlett from cardiac arrest and other doctors assigned to the emergency coronary team had been called. The wildly pulsating line on Bartlett's monitor scope indicated that a failure in the signal system regulating the heart's pace had initiated ventricular tachycardia—a potentially killing rhythm which can rapidly wear out the heart or degenerate into ventricular fibrillation, in which the cardiac muscle twitches ineffectually like a writhing mass of worms. The nurses had already slammed Dr. Bartlett on the chest but when that had not stunned his heart into a healthier rhythm they had administered the prepared bolus of a hundred milligrams of lidocaine and were already into a second dose of pronestyl, another antiarrhythmic, pushed into the bloodstream every two minutes. Margaret Striker remembered afterward saying something like "looks bad" to Jeff Washington without taking her eyes off the monitor where the grim, jerking signal of tachycardia continued unabated. After that the intern and nurse had worked almost wordlessly over their patient while the other nurse rushed to attend another man whose monitor bell had begun its jangling warning call.

In silent concert the nurse and intern proceeded to treat Bartlett, each one anticipating the other's moves and responding to them unhesitatingly as they worked over their now unconscious patient. When the pronestyl had no effect on his tachycardia they moved to precordial shock, setting the voltage first at two hundred watts, then three hundred. But at that point the scope showed a flat line as Bartlett arrested. Instantly the young intern and nurse pushed the level of precordial shock to four hundred. Arcing from the table, Bartlett's body stiffened with the force of the impact as his heart once more began to beat. At that moment the cardiac team—called in such an emergency when there is only three minutes to restart a patient's heart before the brain begins to die—arrived in Bartlett's cubicle. But by then it was clear that Dr. Washington and Margaret Striker had saved him.

Watching Bartlett breathe in that curious moment afterward was something Margaret Striker was to remember long afterward.

After the excitement of the crisis Jeff Washington and Margaret Striker sat in the nursing station, as they had on many previous evenings, watching John Bartlett's scope beat to the steady rhythm of the mechanical pacemaker that had been inserted into his heart to aid it until the trauma of the heart attack had lessened and a decision about the extent of permanent heart blockage could be made. Around them in their cubicles eight persons slept in the silvery dusk like unearthly cyborgs attached to the flickering bedside monitors, unaware that the intern and one of the nurses watching over them were holding hands.

When John Bartlett regained consciousness a day later he had no memory of his brush with death. The moment of the arrest was wiped clean from his mind. But the undeniable evidence of the pacemaker threaded into his heart left no question about the seriousness of its damage. The visible ticking on the monitor scope next to his bed was its mechanical signal, not the natural rhythm of his own heartbeat, and though Bartlett knew he could live a long time in relative health with the aid of a permanent pacemaker implant, it still seemed that overnight, his world had changed. Both the work that had been so compelling and the love that had seemed so promising now appeared beyond his strength.

In the eight days John Bartlett remained in the unit it was plain to his nurse that he was quietly taking accounts with himself. Before the night of his heart attack Bartlett had felt young, virile, and secure, but afterward, when he tried to come to grips with what had happened, he found that he was afraid—afraid to love, afraid to marry a second time, afraid of sex. Margaret Striker knew that this was not an uncommon fear among men who have suffered myocardial infarctions. It was a standing joke that when a man asked his cardiologist if he could have intercourse after a heart attack, the answer was, "With your wife, yes. With your mistress, no," but the story did not seem funny to her when she looked at Bartlett and the woman who loved him. On the night of Bartlett's heart attack Margaret Striker had felt the love between them like a force against his dying, and now it was as if Bartlett was trying to cut the bonds that tied them because he was afraid both for himself and to ask her to take on a life already in jeopardy. Each evening he lay staring at the ceiling of his cubicle, motionless, lost in his own thoughts, as if he was trying to search through memory for some kind of emotional map of his life to indicate where he had been so that he might discover where he was going. Watching him wrestle with his uncertainties, Margaret Striker found herself rummaging through her own emotions, forming questions which suddenly needed answering since the night of Bartlett's arrest, when Jeff Washington had taken her hand. Thus far, she realized, she had framed her world with work. At twenty-three earnestness was her chief quality and it was as if she had put off pleasures for some vague tomorrow when she would have proven her worthiness to enjoy them. It struck her then that she had no idea of who she was—only what: a nurse. Now Jeff Washington seemed to be asking what kind of a woman she might be.

Chapter 8

Two years after her involvement with Jeff Washington had ended Margaret Striker could recall moments from the brief season when their affair had traced spring's coolness into summer's heat with the vividness of Persian miniatures. Scraps from some larger composition that yet held its richness, she remembered flowers in his hands, marigold orange, anemone red and purple, and walks beside him down the cobbled streets of Beacon Hill in spring, his face a vivid sketch in profile beyond when the girl glimpsed the fine old houses with their brass doorknobs, well polished, that somehow had given her an assurance of continuity. And she remembered too what she had felt when he was gone—the loss like a hook bone-deep in her breast; the recollection of that pain still had the force to wound her.

After the first night when Jeff Washington had taken her hand neither had known quite how to deal with their feelings for each other and so they had retreated to the safety of friendship. At first this solution was the simplest. Working in the coronary care unit together, they saw each other constantly and could easily go to lunch together or meet for coffee and, despite the gravity of their responsibilities in the unit, they managed to have fun together and to laugh a great deal even when things went wrong. But after the intern's elective was completed and he moved on to another service Margaret Striker found that she missed him terribly.

Some time after John Bartlett was sent home the nurse received a note from him in which he thanked her and told her he was proceeding with his life as planned. Pleased for him, Margaret Striker had used his letter as an excuse to telephone Jeff Washington and ask him to meet her for lunch. Following her initiative, both managed after that to keep "running into each other" as if by accident. Margaret Striker found herself looking for Jeff Washington wherever she went—in the hospital cafeteria, in the medical library, in the local pub frequented by the interns and nurses after duty, and whenever she found him he would approach her immediately.

In mid-April, after they had begun meeting each other for lunch intentionally with some frequency, Margaret Striker, who had learned what the intern liked to cook, chided him for having neglected to give her a demonstration of his skill, and though he did not respond by inviting her to his apartment for dinner he did bring a pineapple upside-down cake to the unit the next evening. She countered by inviting him to dinner at her small apartment and he came, bearing a bottle of wine and a bunch of flowers. No one had ever brought Margaret Striker either before.

She began cooking for him every other weekend at her apartment and he made dinner for her at his place or they went out somewhere on the alternate weekends, and by skillful planning both managed to have pretty much the same schedules so that they could spend their days off together. As Jeff Washington was making very little money as an intern and Margaret Striker not much more as a nurse, they planned their pleasures carefully, saving money for films and concerts. Both loved music and it became their habit to spend Sunday afternoons together sprawled on pillows on the floor of her living room, listening to the Boston Symphony on the radio and drinking coffee.

Boston itself, both regarded as their special treasure. As spring came on they rented bicycles to explore the old brown city. Both imagined it to be much like London and they began to plan a trip to London together when they both could schedule a month's vacation at the same time.

One balmy day in May they went to Marblehead and rented a sailboat. Margaret Striker, who had always been terrified of the ocean, for reasons she did not fully understand, had been afraid but because she trusted Jeff Washington she had gamely gone along. A tyro at sailing, the intern had managed to capsize the boat in short order and Margaret was pitched into the sea. Thoroughly frightened and soaked when he hauled her out, she was still shaking with cold when they reached her apartment. He had given her a towel rub to warm her up, and so their affair began.

That summer Margaret Striker lived in a world of private intensity and joy she had not known was possible. Everything about Jeff Washington became important to her, the shape of his strong black hands, the depth of his commitment to medicine, the gentle huskiness of his voice. In love completely, Margaret Striker barely thought of Jeff's race in the first weeks of their affair, but slowly she began to realize that what she dismissed was something he could not forget. For while she had quite simply accepted that she was not going to fulfill her mother's expectations in a "proper" marriage, Jeff Washington's ambitions and attitudes all hinged on his blackness, and what did not matter to her mattered fiercely to him. Early in August he was gone. He had received and accepted a fellowship at the National Institute of Health in Washington, D.C.

Margaret Striker saw him on several weekends after he left Boston, until he wrote in September to tell her that he had met someone else—a young woman who was an attorney and was also black. In November she received their wedding announcement.

She went home that weekend for the first time in many months. It was her father who sensed that she was in pain, and without a word he took her in his arms and rocked her as she wept on his shoulder. She could not remember another time in her life he had held her like that. She told him about Jeff then and as she spoke she realized that all that mattered to him was that she was alone again and hurt.

Margaret Striker's first venture into the uncharted territories of her own emotions had left her adrift and shaken. By mid-November she was gone from Boston, back in New York at a new job. That winter she sealed off her memories of Boston in some private realm in the past—like someone closing up a house after there has been a death in it—but in a subtle way the affair with Jeff Washington had changed her. Even as she had become emotionally more vulnerable she had been made more aware of the vulnerability of others, and when she returned to New York, though she intended to continue in coronary care, Margaret Striker was consciously looking for a new direction for herself in nursing. She applied only to institutions that combined a strong reputation for teaching with a commitment to community service, and when no immediate appointment in coronary care had turned up she had taken an assignment as a staff nurse on one of the understaffed medical floors of the hospital where she remained to become a head nurse.

She had expected the job to be an interim one until a place opened up in the hospital's coronary care unit, but it was not long before she discovered that on the busy medical floors more was required of her emotionally and physically than in any previous assignment. For though there was little glory in the staff nurse's job and she found herself once again cast in the role of the physician's handmaiden this no longer seemed to matter much, for she found herself involved with her patients as she had been only rarely since nursing school; when a place opened in the coronary care unit she did not apply for it.

Margaret Striker found an antidote to the solitude of her private life in her profession that first year back in New York. Not only was the spectrum of medicine practiced on the ward broader than it had been in the surgical ICU or in coronary care, but the demands made upon her as a nurse in human terms went deeper. Slowly, in much the same way as a postulant or novice lets herself be drawn into a life dominated by her religious creed, Margaret Striker let herself be drawn into the intense world of the ward. Her days became paced to its rhythms; her friendships were framed upon its society; her rewards were drawn from those rare moments of empathy with her patients when she knew that she had touched another life.

Chapter 9

Margaret Striker had remained a staff nurse on another medical unit for two years before she sought the promotion to become head nurse on 3H, but it took her only a few weeks to discover that her new assignment held more frustration than reward. When she returned to duty on the Monday following the hectic Friday night when Lucille Yaretsky and Mr. Gutzman had been admitted to 3H, she was greeted by a typical post-weekend spate of bad news. Lucille Yaretsky was still alive, but the doctors feared her brain had been damaged extensively, for following her splenectomy she had suffered repeated seizures. Mr. Gutzman was dead. When the surgeons had discovered that his spleen had exploded early on Saturday morning, Teflon had been patched into the ruptured portal vein but his bleeding could not be completely stanched. In the next twenty-four hours, thirty units of whole blood had been poured into him, and when the blood bank's supply was exhausted on Sunday, he had been sustained on plasma. But the vast transfusions, representing the total volume of blood for several individuals that had kept him alive had the ironic side effect of depressing his body's ability to manufacture its own blood supply. When the short-lived platelets in the transfused blood were depleted, he had lost the ability to clot and begun to hemorrhage again. This time, when his heart faltered to a stop in shock, there had been no attempt to resuscitate him. The doctors had gambled on a very slight chance for Mr. Gutzman's life and lost.

Word of his death reached 3H at eight-thirty but had little impact because by then, most of the staff was already too absorbed by several new chapters in the floor's endless melodrama. Almost as soon as the head nurse had returned to the nursing station from report, the emergency room had sent up a seventeen-year-old boy who had swallowed roach powder and lighter fluid after his mother had told him, "Go kill yourself." He had been dragged to the emergency room from the housing project across the avenue by a friend who had seen him collapse and been sent to the unit for stomach lavage and to determine which brand of lighter fluid he had consumed. If the lighter fluid contained naphtha and benzine, it might cause a hemolytic reaction in his bloodstream, dissolving its red blood cells, and whatever fluid he had ingested, the fumes he had inspired could cause severe lung irritation and even pneumonia.

"He smells like a torch," Margaret Striker said, emerging from the room where she and the floor's second assistant resident, Jay Grossman, had been working over the boy's puce-colored body. "He's probably got pneumonia, he seems to be stark-raving mad, and if we don't empty him quickly I swear he'll dissolve!" Tossing a request over her shoulder to the unit clerk, Rosa Perez, she asked her to try to get hold of the boy's mother. "The guys really need to know what this poor kid swallowed," she said as she hurried past the nursing station, pushing a Gomco pump which would be attached to a nasogastric tube for pumping out the boy's stomach, "so try to get his mother in here if you can so we can ask her a few questions."

Within ten minutes the boy's mother came whirling down the hallway like a storm over water, noisily threatening to finish what her son had begun. When the head nurse approached her she began threatening to sue anyone who had lain a finger on her son and, pushing her way past Margaret Striker, she charged into the room where the boy lay, half conscious, and began shouting at him, "You're a failure—a goddamned failure in everything, just like your father," elaborating with a startling variety of obscenities. She was still raging at him an hour later when he was carried away to a psychiatric ward. But by then Margaret Striker was absorbed by the uncomfortable question of who, in error, had managed very nearly to kill eighty-four-year-old Mr. Herbert Bennett on Saturday night.

When she had visited Mr. Bennett's room that morning on rounds he was lying unconscious in his bed like some discarded mechanical toy, a tube stuffed into his mouth and taped in place, breathing noisily as the clicking machine at his bedside pushed his chest up and down. "He was right," Margaret Striker had said grimly, looking down at the frail figure, "people do die here and we seem to be doing our damnedest to be sure one of them will be Herbert Bennett."

When Mr. Bennett had been admitted on Friday Margaret Striker had guessed that he might be a chronic lunger and had cautioned the intern, Eliot Cantor, against prescribing much oxygen for him until the lab readings on his blood gases became available, advice that the intern had taken and the correctness of which was later supported by the lab reports, which showed evidence of a carbon dioxide overload in Mr. Bennett's bloodstream. But on Saturday night someone, observing Mr. Bennett's respiratory troubles, had given him more oxygen than the two liters ordered by nasal cannula—a small snap on nose tube that would mix the tiny flow of oxygen with the room air Mr. Bennett inspired—and when his blood grew richer in oxygen, destroying the only stimulus Mr. Bennett had to breathe, his lungs had simply stopped functioning.

In the crisis Katherine Blaine, the 3H intern on duty that night, had run the tube down his throat into his lungs and attached it to one of the most sophisticated breathing machines in the world,

MA1—a volume pressure respirator that not only forced his lungs to function but with which she could control precisely the amount of oxygen he received. That night she had been trying to maintain his chronic lung mechanism, hoping that he might be quickly weaned from the respirator, for she knew that if Mr. Bennet remained entubated for longer than a few days there was a high risk of irritation that could cause stricture in his throat around the tube, and replacing it with a permanent attachment would require cutting into his windpipe surgically. Monday, however, the question was not so much whether the small man would need a tracheotomy as whether he could ever be separated from a respirator. The doctors now feared that during his respiratory arrest Mr. Bennett might have suffered extensive brain damage.

Investigating what had gone wrong on Saturday night, Margaret Striker soon found that a not unusual series of minor errors had contributed to the one that had nearly killed Mr. Bennett. That evening one of many part-time nurses the hospital had been using to substitute for regular staff in the chronic nursing shortage that afflicted this and every major hospital had been sent to 3H to fill in for Stephanie Forester when she had called in sick. Arriving on the floor at six, the "floater" assumed that all orders for the evening had already been picked up by the charge nurse and relied on the nursing cardex alone for her instructions on Mr. Bennett. She did not realize, therefore, that he was a chronic lunger nor know that intern Eliot Cantor had discontinued the order for oxygen on Mr. Bennett just before he left the floor at three minutes to six after a continuous thirty-three hours on duty. Because the exhausted intern had failed to notify the evening charge nurse of the discontinuance, the order for oxygen stood unchanged in the cardex file and permitted Mr. Bennett "2 liters O2 PRN"—a negligible quantity of oxygen to be administered at the discretion of the nurses.

At about ten o'clock Saturday night, as Mr. Bennett's body rhythms slowed, the accumulated carbon dioxide in his bloodstream had sent his mind wandering restlessly in his sleep. Recognizing his uneasiness as a product of oxygen deprivation, the "floater" had given him pure oxygen—using a malfunctioning wall setup behind his bed and a mask instead of the nasal cannula—unaware that she was saturating his bloodstream with sixty per cent oxygen too quickly. In a nursing note written just before she left the floor at midnight she described him as "sleeping like a baby." But when Mary Obakwanga, the night nurse on change-over rounds, looked in on Mr. Bennett a few minutes later she found that he had stopped breathing. No one knew precisely when, so no one could be sure how extensive Mr. Bennett's brain damage might be until an electroencephalogram was done and Dr. Blaine, acting in the emergency, had simply worked in hope that the respiratory centers of the brain had not been damaged and that Mr. Bennett might be able to survive if he could be carefully weaned from the respirator. On Monday afternoon these chances looked poor.

Mistakes like this were not commonplace. Patients were seldom killed on 3H by nursing or medical error. But they happened. They happened when too many people got overtired or careless. They happened when doctors did not sign off their orders and medications were doubled or given in dangerous sequence or combinations by ignorant nurses. They happened when one shift assumed that another had or had not done a certain job and communications between them broke down or when lab reports went astray or were misfiled or misread and significant facts overlooked that signaled subtle but dangerous patterns developing in a patient. And they also happened when interns miscalculated in their handling of patients, either pushing them into danger by overaggressive treatment or letting them drift into it through their own fear of making decisions.

As head nurse Margaret Striker was expected to review every error to determine if nursing failure was involved, and she shared responsibility for preventing mistakes from happening with the floor's chief resident. And because by far the commonest errors were those, like the one that had nearly killed Mr. Bennett, which originated in confusion about a physician's instructions, the head nurse reviewed every order written by every doctor on every patient on her unit at least three times a day during her nine hours on duty—first as it was transposed from the books used by the doctors to the cardex file used by the nurses, then as it was picked up from the file to be filled by nursing staff, and a third time when she checked off tickets representing medications distributed on her ward and noted them for the physicians to acknowledge by initialing them for entry into the patients' chart records. As tedious as this paper work was for her, the routine provided her with a method of sieving out most potential errors before they could happen and allowed the head nurse to see at a glance which orders needed renewing, which ought to be canceled, and which were questionable. Every order written passed through her hands. Every test requested, every procedure to be implemented, every medication to be given was reviewed by her because as head nurse she was answerable for the performance of her own nurses twenty-four hours a day, seven days a week, and expected to ride herd on the interns and residents to keep any paper mistakes they might make in writing orders from becoming real ones. At the epicenter of the ward's action, her point of vantage was unique and not only permitted the knowledgeable head nurse to judge the strengths and weaknesses of every professional on 3H from the chief resident to the aides but it made her particularly sensitive to any tensions that existed within the staff.

Chapter 10

Margaret Striker was disturbed and frustrated by what had been happening on 3H during her first month in charge. As a staff nurse on a similar medical unit she had formed some very definite notions on how such a ward could and ought to function and the collective mood and attitude of the staff on 3H worried her. Though by and large the clinical work done was rather good most of the time, and under Steve Newman's guidance some of the interns were already becoming remarkably skilled diagnosticians, there was still something so mechanical about the way the staff functioned that the atmosphere on 3H struck the head nurse as about as personal as that of a bus. The patients came and went, a random collection of strangers; their passages were brief and, except for the rare "regulars," like Mr. Desado, whose chronic ailments brought them here rather often or those who stayed on for long periods of time, like Mrs. Teicher, most were scarcely known as individuals. As soon as a bed was empty, it was filled again and in all the coming and going few of the doctors and nurses seemed to find time to be concerned with their patients as anything other than cases.

"Wait'll you see the ascites I've got in 319," one intern might remark to another after admitting an alcoholic whose liver was so damaged that fluids were backing up in his abdominal cavity, blowing it up out of all proportion. Or, "We're getting a marvelous melanoma from New Jersey," or, "That arm in 312 is Gonococcal arthritis," or, "Bet you five to ten your embolectomy ends up a Whipple."

Such remarks, though not unusual in a hospital where teaching and research interests dominated, quite unconsciously betrayed to the head nurse an attitude of detachment among certain of the house staff on 3H that, she was convinced, had helped to create a climate in which errors became more likely because the patients had been rendered all but anonymous. In the past month there had been a series of potentially lethal mistakes made on the ward, the most recent of which had so nearly killed Mr. Bennett. During her first week in charge an evident misreading of an order by one of the staff had resulted in a woman being so overdosed with anticoagulants that she had nearly bled to death, and similar incidents, though far from numerous, had nevertheless followed this first one with an ominous regularity. Diabetics had been left uncontrolled, coronary cases carelessly misjudged, and patients on fluid therapy so mismanaged that they had been driven to the edge of dangerous electrolyte imbalances by the combined clumsiness of certain interns and nurses on enough occasions to be alarming, and almost every day the head nurse could point to some minor incident of carelessness or laziness on the part of a doctor or nurse on the ward. The sloppiness could be explained in part by the exhausting pace the doctors and nurses on 3H were forced to keep. The unit's interns were sometimes on call for forty-eight hours at a stretch and the nurses often worked for fifteen days without a day off, but there was more to the problem than this. Impressed with the notion that they must be cool, functional, and efficient, some of the young interns and residents tended to treat patients as anatomical parts or medical anomalies rather than living individuals, while certain of the nurses were inclined to bury themselves in routine, running through checklists of chores each day, dulled to the needs of their patients in other than physical terms. As a result, much that Margaret Striker considered essential to good nursing and good medical care was missing on her unit and not only were clinical mistakes being made but the instances of psychological neglect were many. It was as if the doctors were so absorbed in proving their mastery of theoretical problems and the nurses so taken up with sheer physical work that, orbiting preoccupied through their own preordained schedules, they had not only begun to lose touch with one another but both were failing to give patients the kind of humane care so many of them desperately needed. But though this state of affairs dismayed the head nurse, she had begun to realize, to her increasing frustration, that despite her own high standards as a nurse there was little she could actually do to improve care on her ward because much of what was wrong on 3H only reflected what was wrong in big-hospital medicine in general and in medical nursing in particular in this and almost every other large urban institution like it in the nation.

For years there had been a shortage of nurses in the United States that had made it difficult for hospitals like this one to recruit enough qualified staff. The shortage had been part of hospital nursing ever since Margaret Striker had graduated from Johns Hopkins in 1968 and had worsened steadily year by year as the supply of nurses nationally began to fall behind demand annually by twenty per cent, producing particularly grave results on the ward services of most big, busy urban medical centers.

In demand everywhere, registered nurses could pick and choose among jobs, and as the quality of life in the center cities deteriorated fewer and fewer new graduates were drawn to ward work even in the most renowned institutions, despite the glaring needs of the patients they served and the greater professional challenges they offered. There were simply too many attractive opportunities elsewhere professionally, both in specialized hospital units like the intensive care sections, where the pay and the staffing ratios were better, or in research specialties like anaerobic and hyperbaric nursing, or outside the big hospitals altogether, in public health and independent practice, for general service nursing in big city hospitals to be able to recruit and hold enough qualified nurses. As registered nurses browsed from one green pasture to the next professionally, creating an exodus from hospital nursing that reached critical proportions by the early 1970s, the quality of care within the major hospitals declined steadily. As staffing worsened situations like the one on 3H became typical not of the worst but of the best hospitals.

Faced with continuing attrition, as the line between "safe" and "unsafe" staffing was approached, some of the most reputable hospitals had accelerated their recruitment overseas. But just as RNs from all over the English-speaking world who could pass the licensure examinations began to flood into the United States—most enlisted for service in the center-city hospitals—administrators faced with soaring costs in these same institutions took the course of chopping nursing staff budgets to recoup deficits so that many unfilled vacancies on the wards became "unbudgeted vacancies," jobs that existed in need but not in fact. It was a move that had the unhappy effect of guaranteeing that there would be no improvement in a situation in which the best-staffed wards in most urban hospitals were being run with about half the ideal number of nurses required and the worst-staffed wards with a third or less, assuring and producing an even more rapid turnover among the nurses who still opted for such service so that it became unusual for them to stay in their grueling jobs for more than a year at a stretch.

When Margaret Striker had come to 3H she had nine registered nurses, two licensed practical nurses, and four aides to staff the forty-two-bed unit round the clock seven days a week—a number soon to be reduced by resignations to just about half of that considered adequate to meet the floor's needs. Her staff was ranked beneath her in a scheme of organization Florence Nightingale had modeled on the British Army, which placed the head nurse in a position roughly equivalent to that of a master sergeant on her ward. Margaret Striker was expected to oversee the work of her nurses and aides and coordinate it with the orders of the physicians on 3H in much the same way that a master sergeant fulfills the commands of officers by delegating authority downward through the ranks. Theoretically this scheme reinforced a chain of command that accorded superior status, responsibility, and pay to those with superior credentials and experience, but on 3H equal rank did not equal nurses make and Margaret Striker knew that there was more diversity than uniformity in her mismatched staff and little or no unity among them as a result.

The four aides were from the West Indies and Puerto Rico, one of the two LPNs was an immense Polish girl from Buffalo and the other a black from New York, and the registered nurses were about equally divided between American and foreign-born, with representatives from Rwanda, the Philippines, India, and Jamaica West Indies teamed with Americans whose accents bespoke the South, Northeast, Midwest, Puerto Rico, and New York's Harlem —a mixture that for all its cultural and linguistic charm was flawed by educational, ethnic, and racial differences that lay beneath the surface of the group's relationships like a fault line, the source of hidden strains that threatened to split them into quarreling factions.

All of these elements, short staffing, racial friction, and the irritability that came with overwork, had plagued the nursing staff before Margaret Striker had come to 3H and the new head nurse could do nothing to change this. She was still routinely having to ask her staff to rotate from days to evenings and nights to cover the wards' needs round the clock seven days a week, and there was no let up in the requirement that they each jam the equivalent of seventy hours of patient care into each forty-hour work week simply to maintain safe standards on the unit. But the extraordinary demands that were made on the floor's nurses did not end here, for the chores attached to advanced medicine of the kind practiced in this teaching hospital had multiplied. Nursing had found itself being asked to take on all the extra little odd jobs no one else wanted—most of which, though they had little to do with patient care, if left undone would have amounted to neglect. Hence, simply to keep the unit running the nurses on 3H were, in addition to carrying a double load of patient duty, required to count and stack the linens, sort out infectious garbage, move the furniture, accompany patients in wheelchairs and on stretchers about the hospital whenever the unionized "transport" workers were off duty, wipe up the floors when the unionized housekeepers went home, haul heavy supplies about, fix machines when electricians went home, keep track of the floor's pharmacy, pick up after the doctors, answer the telephones, count the narcotics, pass out and pick up the meal trays, and bundle up the dirty linens— all without any increment in a pay scale that saw most of them earning something in the vicinity of ten thousand dollars a year— a sum all of them knew could be matched by nurses on private duty, who picked their own hours and cases and avoided most of the menial chores that had been foisted on the staff nurses. Misused as maids of all work, driven relentlessly to try to keep even minimal standards through endless rounds of routine which were obdurately the same despite the continuing drama of life and death on the ward, many of the nurses on 3H had found their commitment to nursing slowly eroding, and some of them, Margaret Striker was aware, were rapidly losing the will to carry on. It was a syndrome the head nurse was too familar with, one that she had seen destroy many good nurses in the past, and one she had experienced herself at the beginning of her professional career. First, she knew, came exhaustion, then a sense of the pointlessness of continuing to struggle against an endless tide of problems, and finally from the anger that grew out of professional frustration came depression and the death of caring. To survive emotionally on 3H Margaret Striker knew that both she and her nurses would need to have restored to them a sense of professional pride and esprit if they were ever to magic out of what was essentially a brutalizing experience, a rebirth of the compassion that would sustain them. For it took a special kind of stamina to continue to do, day after day with too few hands, all the ugly, sad, hopeless little chores that were part of the care of the very sick, and a special kind of determination would be needed, Margaret Striker realized, to keep high standards of care enforced on a floor where it seemed that every day the nurses' work became more fragmented and thankless.

Chapter 11

There was no way the head nurse could take the pressure implied by their limited numbers off her staff. That much was as certain as that Mr. Desado—who was sent home in the last week of August, a cheerful Lazarus quite incredulous that he had once more made it by death's door—would be back again. A stream of admissions followed a stream of discharges. Mrs. Teicher, brave in a blue dress, also was sent "home," to the nursing facility where she lived. The two heart patients, Lee and Nelson, were successfully regulated on digitalis and released, as was Mr. James, the cellist who won a second remission from acute leukemia, a "miracle" he celebrated by waltzing the head nurse breathlessly around the lounge. Moments like this brightened Margaret Striker's days and the clinical "victories" on 3H outstripped the losses, but though the faces of the patients changed, the overall mood of the ward did not and the head nurse knew that despite the increasing easiness of her own associations with Eliot Cantor and Kate Blaine among the interns, and Bill Fischer, the assistant resident, there was still a cold distance between most of the nurses and the doctors on 3H that needed to be bridged.

There was of course some explanation for the particularly strained situation among the staff on 3H in what had happened between Margaret Striker's predecessor and the then newly appointed chief resident when Steve Newman had first come to 3H in July with five new interns in tow. At that time, Margaret Striker had been told, the previous head nurse had already been at the end of her professional tether and was on the verge of resigning. In her last months in charge she had let things on the ward slide badly, permitting her own frustration to communicate itself to her staff, reinforcing their professional dissatisfactions and legitimizing the anger of those nurses in particular who blamed the doctors for their professional misuse. When Newman had arrived on ward he had found himself facing a quietly hostile nursing staff, many of whom were not only professionally unhappy but racial and feminist militants as well. Not one to handle such a situation diplomatically, Newman, an outspoken fellow very conscious of his newly gained authority as chief resident, had reacted by scoffing at the nurses' grievances, and after making it quite clear that he had little interest in their problems he had withdrawn with his staff of interns and assistant residents into a kind of psychological fastness no nurse had since been permitted to enter. It was a reaction which, though partly justified, had done little to improve an already bad situation, and though Margaret Striker recognized that it was up to her to reopen a dialogue with the chief resident she did not know quite how to approach him.

Steve Newman was no easy person for Margaret Striker to reckon with. She had known the chief resident both as an intern and an assistant resident when he had been assigned to the ward on which she had worked as a staff nurse and she had watched his metamorphosis from a fledgling doctor to his present eminence with mixed emotions, for in many ways it seemed to her that Dr. Newman embodied what was best and what was worst in the ethos of this hospital.

Short and round with an improbable Fu Manchu mustache, the

chief resident was a theatrical young man who conducted the medical business of the ward in a highly personal way, combining an icy diagnostic brilliance with a maverick style that struck the more conventional head nurse as slightly outrageous. With little respect for propriety and virtually no bedside manner, Newman maneuvered his way through the daily rounds of the unit with the *chutzpah* of a New York delicatessen waiter—cheerfully insulting his interns, the nurses, and all but the sickest patients with a fine disregard for propriety.

"Well, well, well, Mrs. Katz," he once greeted a woman soon to be discharged, "so you're going home? Congratulations! You're the second one to walk out of here in a month. My interns and the nurses tried hard to kill you, but I wouldn't let them." When advised by another patient to see a doctor for a heavy head cold Newman responded: "I would, but there's no one in this hospital I'd trust to examine me."

Dr. Newman explained his antic irreverence as "the only appropriate response possible to an absurd proposition"—the responsibility he had been given as a chief resident of simultaneously initiating five inexperienced interns into the delicate arts of diagnosis and treatment on a ward in which many of the patients' illnesses made them particularly vulnerable to mishandling. And for all the hyperbole of Newman's humor, the chief resident meant exactly what he said. A skilled practitioner himself, Steve Newman had few illusions about the perfectibility of hospitals or physicians in general and because he was in charge on 3H he was particularly aware of the clumsiness of his newly hatched brood of five interns. He took his duty of trying to turn them into competent physicians very seriously indeed.

Unlike many of the other chief residents in medicine, Newman was not an Ivy League product. He had come up to win an appointment at this renowned hospital out of Brooklyn public schools and a state university and, proud of his achievements, he flaunted his lack of blue ribbon credentials. Mirroring the brash qualities of his home city in both his irreverent style and his taste for success, Newman made no apologies for the fact that he was out one day for a share in the spoils of New York's big time medical action and hoped eventually to combine a high-powered practice in cardiology with a research and teaching appointment in a hospital like this one. For besides the rewards of money, status, and power that went with such a career, Steve Newman was interested in Medicine for its own sake, and for all his cockiness he was, in fact, a True Believer; medicine was a passion he had pursued since boyhood and he was unquestioningly committed to its long quarrel with mortality.

But, watching the chief resident in action, Margaret Striker had a queasy feeling, for despite a warmth that lurked beneath Steve Newman's raffish manner that compelled him to pat old ladies in their wheelchairs whenever he breezed by them, Dr. Newman's fascination with the arcane arts of Medicine made him too aggressive in his tactics on 3H for Margaret Striker's tastes. Though perhaps better than anyone else on the ward the head nurse could understand the pressures on the chief resident, for in the uneven record of her order books she could read a profile of the strengths and weaknesses of each of his interns, it often seemed to her that Steve Newman placed such emphasis on developing the analytic skills of these five that he neglected the human needs of his patients. And though Margaret Striker realized that it was as much the chief resident's job to prepare his interns for the future as to cope with the ward in day-to-day terms, there were moments when Newman's enthusiastic teaching methods could turn the pursuit of a medical answer in a complex case into a kind of trophy hunt, introducing an element of rivalry into the practice of medicine on 3H that gave it a curiously athletic quality. It was the whiff of the arena on the 3H that set Margaret Striker at odds with Dr. Newman, for she suspected that in many ways the chief resident regarded the care of the sick as the ultimate sport, a game of wits to be played against the wiliest of opponents, death, in which he was determined to prove himself a star performer.

Chapter 12

The long Labor Day weekend had been tranquil. It almost seemed as if, insisting on the last pleasures of summer, people had been deciding not to be ill. The ward's census was down by four for the first time in forty days and Margaret Striker and Marie Velasquez, comparing notes on Tuesday morning, hardly dared remark on the floor's peacefulness for fear of tempting fate. Both were, quite frankly, superstitious. They insisted that on medical floors like 3H holidays produced quiet times which were followed by stormy ones—that there were always more crises at the full of the moon, and that whenever trouble did begin to erupt on the ward it followed a pattern of threes. One heart attack begot two more; one death almost always presaged another pair within the week. And indeed, this Tuesday morning quiet was one of expectation—3H was in line for the next admission through the emergency room and Kate Blaine was already downstairs patrolling the ER to see what prize the city's lottery of griefs might turn up.

It produced Dela Hanze and when Margaret Striker took the call from Dr. Blaine announcing her arrival she wondered aloud if the intern would even get her new patient upstairs alive. Eighty years old, already in a deep coma with the acid-base balance of her blood lethally deranged as a result of diabetes and chronic kidney failure, Mrs. Hanze, from the description Dr. Blaine had given, was only minutes away from death. Reacting almost by reflex in the emergency, the head nurse paged Dr. Newman to notify the chief resident of the imminent arrival of a crisis case, and then began getting ready for the probability of a code 700 being called. The 700 code was used to page members of an emergency team from wherever they might be in the hospital whenever a cardiac emergency occurred, and when one was called as many as a dozen doctors and several extra nurses might be brought dashing to assist in what was almost invariably a frenzied attempt to save a life in the fractional interlude of three minutes, the time between when the heart stopped beating and the moment cell death began in the brain, producing irreversible damage.

In such a situation every drug the doctors could conceivably call for needed to be ready at the nurses' fingertips on the crash cart, the mobile unit used in cardiac emergencies on which all the drugs and devices that might be required to assist a dying heart were prestocked, and Margaret Striker, who more than once in her nursing career had seen a jagged line of light on a monitor slump into a flat line that signaled death because something had gone amiss in the middle of a 700 code, had a habit of mistrusting everyone and of checking to see that the crash cart was in perfect order when there was no expectation of a code 700 in the offing.

By the time the stretcher bearing the unconscious Mrs. Hanze came rattling down the corridor, with Kate Blaine and Steve Newman trotting alongside, the chief resident firing questions at the wide-eyed intern as they ran toward room 320, everything was in readiness. Margaret Striker had already hung the intravenous fluids she knew Newman would call for to carry medication directly into Mrs. Hanze's bloodstream at her bedside. The crash cart stood waiting outside the door and as the stretcher swung into the room the head nurse was assembling for Newman's and Blaine's immediate use premeasured doses of alkali and soda bicarbonate normally used in the emergency treatment of acidosis and associated chemical imbalances of the blood that can have devastating effects on the heart.

Mrs. Hanze's breath was coming in rasping gasps that sounded like someone tearing cloth as they rolled her off the stretcher and the head nurse pushed a portable electrocardiograph machine into place next to the bed. Immediately the 3H team was at work. As the head nurse began taping the ECG terminals in place Ellen King, the staff nurse Margaret Striker had assigned to Mrs. Hanze, slapped an oxygen mask over her face. The chief resident and the intern, one on each side of the bed, bent over the unconscious Mrs. Hanze, probing for usable veins for the IV implants in her arms and legs. Only one was in place when Margaret Striker,

70

who was by then running a test strip on the ECG to be sure that it was functioning properly, reported in a tight voice, "She's wide on the QRS, Steve—or so it looks to me—way wide and tent-shaped T-waves. . . ."

In an instant the chief resident stood over the electrocardiograph machine, studying the eccentric record of Mrs. Hanze's heartbeat being scrawled out. In the exaggerated configuration of lines that followed the first jagged indicator of Mrs. Hanze's atrial heartbeat he read an ugly message: Mrs. Hanze's heart was staggering toward standstill, probably poisoned by an overload of potassium in her blood that had resulted from a failure of her kidneys to function properly. He began snapping out orders in a voice that was very low, calling his shots from the ECG like a man directing artillery. Margaret Striker responded, flicking the tops off the premeasured glass vials with a snapping motion of her fingertips and withdrawing their contents into syringes, which she handed to Katherine Blaine to administer or injected herself into the "piggyback" join that allowed the drugs to mix with the intravenous fluid.

"Hit her with fifty units of insulin," Newman barked, "and get in another line for glucose fast."

Katherine Blaine began probing a vein in Mrs. Hanze's ankle that had popped up below an elastic tourniquet Ellen King had wrapped in place, slapping at it with her fingers as she fished for it with a needle while Margaret Striker worked at Newman's unsuccessful implant in the woman's arm.

"Do you want a code called?" she asked the chief in a flat, commandingly quiet voice as she worked. "And do you want me to get a CVP line ready for you?"

"No code yet . . . Get that vein up instead of CVP . . . not time . . ." Newman murmured, bending over the ECG tape, preoccupied, watching the printout. "Christ, bicarb . . . now . . ." Newman commanded just as Kate Blaine hit home with a butterfly needle and Margaret Striker handed her an IV line to fix in place.

"How much?" the head nurse quizzed in a cold voice, already

breaking the top of two hundred milliequivalents of intravenous sodium bicarbonate. "One, two, three hundred?" She handed Dr. Blaine the syringe of two hundred as Newman looked up, his face still frozen in a look of concentration. "Come on, Margaret—you know," he growled. "Two hundred, of course." "I might know, Steve, but what if I didn't? It's a bad habit. . . ." The air crackled for the fraction of a moment and then without comment Newman looked back at the ECG. "Now give her two grams of calcium gluconate."

They kept working; commands were snapped out, hands flew, and there was grace and discipline evident in the unison of their efforts. But the silence in the room, punctuated only by Newman's barked orders, became taut as Mrs. Hanze's irregular Cheyne-Stokes breathing pattern persisted, indicating continuing heart failure. Newman, concentrating on the ECG, did not look up. Then Margaret Striker, her ears keyed for change in Mrs. Hanze's respiration, suddenly smiled. "She's coming back, Steve," she said as the rhythm switched subtly toward a more normal pattern. "She's coming back and congratulations, Doctors."

"Well done yourself, Nurse" growled Newman, not looking up from the ECG printout, where he had already read the good news that Mrs. Hanze would live. "Wanna see?" He gesticulated, holding up the ECG strip like a banner. "Close as hell, but a good job did it. . . ."

Mrs. Hanze moaned. In what seemed like an almost miraculous response her ash-white color began to pink, her breath became less and less labored, and within a few minutes Newman, still standing over the ECG, reported with satisfaction that her heartbeat had begun to stabilize in a normal rhythm.

"But the electrolytes will need watching constantly, ladies," he said to the head nurse and intern Kate Blaine simultaneously. "So let's see what you liberated wenches can manage with this one." He tore off a section of ECG tape for Mrs. Hanze's chart record, dropped the rest of it on the floor, gave Margaret Striker's arm a light pinch and walked out of the room, leaving the head nurse, Dr. Blaine, and Ellen King to straighten up Mrs. Hanze's bloodied bed and pick up the debris that had accumulated in the crisis. It was a calculated, teasing performance that left the three women shaking their heads and smiling ruefully.

That day, following the unwritten rule of three, there were two more emergencies on the ward. At midmorning one of the several leukemics on the floor began spiking high, uncontrollable fevers that indicated the possible onset of sepsis—a systemic infection that becomes rampant when the body's defenses are severely depressed—and just after noon a new admission was brought in, bleeding uncontrollably from an ulcer that had perforated. In each instance the chief resident and head nurse worked in concert with the cool precision of the seasoned professionals they were and managed to beat back death, and when it was all over both shone with the special exhilaration of their efforts.

Steve Newman, sassy, theatrical, and difficult, was both exasperating and exciting to work with and yet dependable in crisis situations. Despite her ambivalent feelings toward him, Margaret Striker grudgingly admired this chief resident. The machismo element that had been evident in his performance with Mrs. Hanze, his sarcastic attitude toward the particular interns Margaret Striker most admired for their gentleness, Eliot Cantor and Kate Blaine, even Newman's condescending treatment of her own nurses and overaggressiveness in the handling of certain patients could not cancel the fact that the chief resident was a superbly talented practitioner, bold and calculating in situations of high risk. She knew that his decisiveness in emergencies like the one with Mrs. Hanze was matched by an intuitive diagnostic skill that was impressively in evidence at chart rounds—the private reviews Newman held with his interns off the floor several mornings a week—and whenever Margaret Striker attended these sessions she felt the same addictive excitement watching Newman in action as a theoretician that she experienced working with him in a crisis out on the ward.

Dr. Newman's performances at chart rounds were dazzling. Like a juggler able to keep countless objects in the air simultaneously, he had an uncanny knack for keeping track of thousands of pieces of information about the unit's forty-two patients and seemed always to know how each intern was getting on with every case. Alternately wheedling and sarcastic, Newman would put the five through medical hoops in the privacy of his chart rounds and he made it worrisome for any intern who fell behind the pack in the chase for medical answers on difficult cases. Attacking them wherever they were vulnerable, he saved his worst scorn for those who vacillated, like the head nurse's friend Eliot Cantor, and in the rivals game for status and future appointments at this hospital, which were very much a part of the hidden agenda on 3H, the chief resident's displeasure meant a loss of points.

Newman's insistence that his interns keep up with the newest medicine was understandable, for in his chart rounds the chief resident was principally concerned with preparing the five for the future rather than with coping with patients' needs in the present, and since much of the work of this research and teaching hospital was aimed at finding the biological keys to unresolved diseases and developing techniques to prolong life, there was a heavy research emphasis in Newman's orientation of his interns. There were few compassionate niceties about the patients at chart rounds. The chief resident made it clear that the interns were to regard 3H as a living textbook in medicine and that they were to learn to use their intellects to analyze their patients' diseases in much the same way surgical interns learned to use their knives. Anyone admitted to the ward was to be approached with complete detachment. His symptoms were to be analyzed and the most intimate facts about his physical and emotional state laid out before the group at chart rounds like a patient etherized upon a table. For hidden in a welter of confusing fragments of information, Newman knew, the elusive shape of death might lie unseen, and it was his job to teach his inexperienced staff to discern its forms.

Because many patients referred to this hospital were those whose complicated or mysterious ailments had baffled other physicians, Newman's staff often faced formidable problems in diagnosis, and the sharp edge of rivalry he encouraged among them had its uses. Under his leadership chart rounds became problem-

74

solving exercises in which the interns and residents competed with Newman to analyze complex cases and design model strategies for treatment which employed the most advanced theory, technique, and gadgetry. And though the head nurse often shuddered to think of the effects the pursuit of some abstruse medical answer might produce for the hapless patient involved, as a knowledgeable spectator who had watched many physicians perform she recognized Steve Newman as a master of the arts of medicine.

Yet even when a diagnosis was made on 3H, treatment could be subtle and difficult and the young doctors under Newman often found themselves engaged in delicate balancing acts when they began fiddling with the intricately interrelated systems on which life depends. Chronic cardiac patients, for instance, could become so sensitive to digitalis—the drug most commonly used to strengthen a weakened heart—that the slightest miscalculation in dosage could send them spinning into dangerous arrhythmias that duplicated those which occur in the aftermath of a heart attack. Leukemics, like the one who had nearly gone into sepsis on the day of Mrs. Hanze's admission, faced awesome risks during the dangerous interval when the poisons used in chemotherapy to kill off cancer cells crowding out healthy ones in their bone marrow also wiped out their defenses against any bacteria or fungus they might harbor in their bodies, even those common in everyone's mouth and intestinal tract. And besides the drugs with direct toxic effects, many routinely employed on 3H had indirect but dangerous side-effects. Diuretics, used too aggressively, could derange the subtle electrolyte balances that fine tune the physiology and produce complicated and lethal results; certain antibiotics used almost as commonly as aspirin could, in massive dosages, destroy the auditory nerve endings in the inner ear, causing deafness and a total loss of balance. Other drugs precipitated preleukemic states and certain tranquilizers had also been implicated in producing blood dyscrasias. Even the steroids—used with great success to depress slow-growing cancers and thus to lengthen life—could so mask opportunistic secondary infections that until these became murderously rampant they went undetected and unchecked.

Each disease had its field of interractions and presented hypothetical questions that needed consideration before they became troublesome realities. Each drug had its surprise couplings. Each combination of medical moves entailed a combined set of hazards. And while the young doctors on 3H were engaged in their gambler's game of finely calculated risks, their insights into the body's responses to their incursions into its mysterious balances were dependent on fragmentary clues they fetched up through testing. Sometimes they seemed to Margaret Striker like fishermen on the edge of some vast ocean trying to understand the ecology of the depths from evidence their nets dragged from the surfaces, for even as they garnered proofs of progress against certain diseases, they knew that their knowledge was partial and that for all the immense learning of their profession they were confronted by its practical limitations on 3H every day.

Chapter 13

Julian Berman, a shambling ghost of a man with a face like a crumpled piece of paper, was a walking, articulate reminder of the doctor's limitations. The ward's resident "madman," he stalked the halls wrapped in a blanket he fancied as a dressing gown, loudly warning other patients and visitors alike against "the fools, incompetents, and pretenders here who call themselves doctors," and though seldom hostile to Margaret Striker or the other nurses he had recently bounced a slight lady hematologist off the walls of 3H as if she were a handball and had twice threatened to throttle Frank Richards, the intern in charge of his case.

Mr. Berman's disgruntlement with doctors in general was understandable. He had come to the ward in July, after having spent more than a year going from hospital to hospital and doctor to doctor in search of some explanation for a bizarre malaise that periodically sent him into states of psychosis in which he systematically smashed up his wife and house while calling for the police.

When admitted to 3H he trailed a history of inconclusive diagnoses in a chart record the size of a city phonebook. But though every doctor who had seen Mr. Berman was convinced that his madness was organically based—and Steve Newman and his interns had for weeks pursued an answer in the puzzling case with all the enthusiasm of a pack of Englishmen riding to hounds—they had succeeded only in eliminating a long list of possible diseases that could cause dementia and had not yet arrived at a conclusive diagnosis. And Mr. Berman—who at one point had slipped from madness into stupor and near-death before spontaneously recovering his present precarious state, in which periods of cagey sanity alternated with periods of equally cagey insanity—consequently had decided to refuse any further investigation of his body by knife, needle, syringe, enema, or X-ray.

"I can't think any of 'em know what they're looking for anymore," he complained bitterly to Margaret Striker in one of his saner moments when the head nurse had come to plead with him to submit to still another series of gastrointestinal proddings, "and they'd gladly kill me at this point just to satisfy their curiosity!"

But despite the weight of contrary opinion stacked against him in Mr. Berman's case history and sheaves of tests which showed that his patient's liver was normal, Steve Newman did know what he was looking for. The chief resident was convinced that Mr. Berman's episodic insanity indicated hepatic disease and by mid-August, when it had seemed that diagnosis in the case was as remote as it had been on the day of Mr. Berman's admission, he had called in a specialist recognized as an expert on the liver to consult on the case.

A principal site for the detoxification of the blood and the conversion of food proteins into plasma proteins, the liver plays a decisive but still not entirely understood role in the biochemistry of the brain. In rare cases, shifts in blood chemistry caused by its malfunctioning could result in psychiatric changes of the kind Mr. Berman had exhibited without producing other definitive symptoms. Though Newman could find only the sketchiest indications that Berman's liver was in trouble, he decided neverthe-

77

less to pursue his hunch that an occult hepatitis had slowly been destroying Mr. Berman's liver even though no signs of tissue destruction had emerged from several biopsies.

Taking the conflicting test results to one of the senior physicians at the hospital who was a specialist in hepatic problems, Newman reviewed Berman's case with him. He emphatically supported the chief resident's impression and suggested that Berman at once be put on a controlled diet used when there has been extensive damage to the liver to see if lowering his protein and carbohydrate intake might not improve his mental state. He also advised one more needle biopsy be performed.

Two days later Mr. Berman had begun to bleed internally in quantity sufficient for the dissolved product to stain his urine dark red, and his irritability had increased noticeably. In that week alone he tossed off the walls the lady doctor who had approached him for a blood sample, twice threatened Frank Richards with mayhem, and sent his wife wailing from the ward after loudly accusing her of trying to murder him.

Shaking a bony finger in warning, a baleful look in his pale blue eyes, Mr. Berman had repeatedly insisted to Margaret Striker and anyone else who would listen that his wife wanted him dead. But whenever the head nurse had talked with the bewildered Mrs. Berman she had been impressed both by the woman's anxiety about the doctor's lack of progress with her husband and by her very real concern for him. "My God, he's suffering so," she had confided to the head nurse one day at the end of August. "I can't bring him any bad news that will add to his troubles. But the bills, bills, bills! You wouldn't believe the bills. We may lose our house, everything my poor husband worked so hard for, and no one can even tell me why! Will he never be well? What if there's nothing left for him to go home to? What will become of us?"

The longer the doctors had remained baffled, the greater Mrs. Berman's tension had become. After her husband had begun his mysterious hemorrhaging she seemed to Margaret Striker almost to change visibly. Once rather elegant—despite an expression of perpetual worry—Mrs. Berman now wore the disheveled look of

someone whose life has become entirely and unexpectedly un-
raveled and after Dr. Richards told her he intended to abandon
the special liver diet she became so nervous that whenever she
used lipstick the trembling of her hand made her misapply it in a
way that gave her mouth a blurred, uncertain aspect that, combined with her lusterless eyes, made Margaret Striker wonder
aloud whether Mrs. Berman was not now relying on a dangerous
combination of pills and alcohol to keep herself going. But when
the head nurse expressed to Dr. Richards her growing concern
for Mrs. Berman the intern, evidently preoccupied, seemed to take
little notice of what she said and she was left to cope with Mrs.
Berman's disintegration in whatever way she chose.

It was not the first time the head nurse had found herself trying
to pick up the pieces of someone else's fractured life on 3H. Dealing with the families of patients on the ward was very much a part
of nursing's responsibility, especially as there were several in the
ward's present complement of doctors who had a way of skirting
the emotional issues on a given case by concentrating on the medical ones. All too often, sitting quietly behind the nursing station
picking up orders, Margaret Striker had overheard one or another
of these doctors deliver some painful notice to an anxious family
in the toneless manner of a newscaster giving a bulletin about a
catastrophe in some remote place and then seen him walk away before his stunned audience could recover enough to respond.

Sometimes the "doctor's brushoff" was necessary; anxious family members—demanding explanations or attention and service
for their loved ones that could only be matched in a luxury
hotel—often did waste the doctors' *and* the nurses' time and try
their tempers when more pressing problems were before them.
But at the opposite end of the spectrum some of the young doctors, preoccupied with their own very specific interests, could un-
wittingly be quite callous, not because they were heartless but because they were literally insensitive. The same facts which a
worried husband or wife could find utterly terrifying were commonplace to the doctors, and because they dealt with chronic
reality of serious illness every day they were sometimes quite

unable to comprehend the impact their words could have on their uninformed listeners. More often than not in such a situation it fell to one of the 3H nurses or to Margaret Striker herself to try to provide answers for the ageless questions people ask when they begin to face the possibility that someone they love may be dying. "How can this be?" Margaret Striker had heard people ask in a hundred different ways. "What shall we do now?" "Do I dare hope?" "How long can he live?" "What will become of me?" And when the head nurse listened to the harassed Mrs. Berman she knew that once again these questions needed answering.

But when she sought out Frank Richards to ask the intern what he planned next for Mr. Berman and how soon he would do the recommended liver biopsy, so that the next time Mrs. Berman confronted her in the hallway with her eyes full of fear she might give the terrified woman some rational answers, the head nurse was stunned by the young doctor's response. "No biopsy," he said flatly. "No biopsy because he could begin hemorrhaging again." Then, his face solemn, he asked her with perfect seriousness, "Has it occurred to you, Margaret, that Mrs. Berman may have been trying to kill her husband quietly right here on 3H? That the old nut is right, that she wants him dead? . . . I won't biopsy that liver because I'm now convinced Dr. Newman is right, but for the wrong reasons; Berman's liver is involved. It's being destroyed by slow, methodical poisoning!" Startled, the head nurse laughed, but when she thought about Dr. Richards' outlandish suggestion later she could not reject it entirely. Something of an expert in plasma protein metabolism as a result of her work in the surgical research unit back at the beginning of her career in nursing, Margaret Striker had all along been privately persuaded, as was Dr. Newman, that Mr. Berman's liver was at the source of his troubles and when the test regimen limiting his diet had not produced results, the head nurse had been surprised.

But now, considering Dr. Richards' suggestion that intentional poisoning might have caused a slow, insidious destruction of Mr.

80

Berman's liver and resulted in his sporadic insanity and recent hemorrhage, the notion made a kind of grim sense to her that also explained Mrs. Berman's anxiety. And though still unconvinced, that evening Margaret Striker asked her nurses to put Mrs. Berman under constant surveillance whenever she was on the ward and to keep a record of anything she might be giving her husband to eat or drink. The head nurse also decided that the next day she would sit in on chart rounds to see if Dr. Richards had the courage of his convictions.

An ambitious and gifted intern with a firm grasp of the competitive realities of hospital life, Richards, a born showman, loved drama in any situation, particularly when it attached to his patients and could be used to draw attention to himself. Even in normal situations he was able to convey an air of urgency in whatever he did and to give the impression that every case he handled was more difficult and compelling than those to which his fellow interns were assigned. Dr. Richards enjoyed nothing more than to show off at chart rounds by leading his colleagues on some fine and fascinating chase after a clever medical theory. And because Mr. Berman had mystified him for too long he did not intend to miss this opportunity for making up his losses by giving a rousing performance.

Bouncing on his heels, his head inclined at an angle, Richards began by marshaling chapter and verse to prove his new theory that Mrs. Berman was deliberately trying to murder her husband. "Everything points to it," he argued, his arms thrown wide in the gesture of a Texas trial lawyer, his glasses perched on the tip of his nose. "The blood product spilling into his urine last week was a final proof of extensive tissue breakdown—I tell you, some-*one*, not some*thing*, is killing Mr. Berman."

"Did you biopsy the liver, Frank?" Newman interrupted in a reedy voice he reserved for occasions when his favorite intern was getting out of hand. "I wanted you to biopsy his liver."

"Steve," the intern instructed his superior, pulling himself to his full six-foot height over the short, round chief resident and looking down on him, the scholar instructing the fool, "you know a needle biopsy is contraindicated if the liver is grossly damaged. The blood product in the urine could be a final manifestation of necrosis and if it is the liver that's heavily involved, he might hemorrhage on biopsy. . . ."

"Biopsy the liver, Richards," the chief resident retorted, glaring up at the intern, "or you'll find out if this latest theory was correct with a post-mortem."

Three days afterward, the liver biopsy was returned with a reading of "acute viral hepatitis with extensive necrosis." Mr. Berman's liver was all but dead. That same day the doctors also learned, through Margaret Striker, that Mrs. Berman had been regularly sneaking chocolate cakes to her husband—even, as it turned out, during the period in which his diet had been officially controlled to test for liver malfunction. As the undetected hepatitis had progressed over the past year, Mr. Berman had become less and less able to handle a normal diet. Whenever he ate richly the overload of carbohydrates and proteins literally became poison to him, tipping his brain into toxic states that resulted in episodic insanity. The many needle biopsies, by a fluke, had evidently drawn tissue from one section of the liver unaffected by its progressive disease until the last. Thrown off the pursuit of hepatitis on repeated occasions, the many doctors who had seen Mr. Berman had compiled a history that at first made it almost embarrassing for the callow 3H team to challenge the record. But as the slow destruction of his liver continued and Mr. Berman's mental disorders increased, so also had his general disability, producing symptoms so diffuse that his primary disease had become masked by its secondary effects and was made more difficult to discern.

Chapter 14

"How'd Mrs. Berman take the news?" Eliot Cantor asked, setting a tray down opposite Margaret Striker at lunch the next day in the hospital cafeteria.

"She told me about her nephew Myron," the head nurse replied, extracting a sandwich from a crumpled paper bag. "It seems Myron had hepatitis and recovered, so she found it hard to understand why Mr. Berman wasn't going to get better." She hesitated, thinking about what in fact had been a tearful scene as the stunned Mrs. Berman had tried to grapple with the news that her husband, at fifty-six, probably had only a year or two to live. "And then she asked how everybody could have missed such a simple diagnosis for a whole year. . . ."

"Seems like a legitimate question," Cantor replied unhappily. "*We'd* like to know ourselves how we missed it for ten weeks. . . . Geez," he mused, gloomily poking at what looked like a pop-art version of a salad on his plate; it featured plastic-looking tomatoes next to equally plastic-looking rolls of turkey and bologna. "We *did* check liver function routinely when he was admitted and the enzymes showed nothing," he continued, explaining as much to himself as to Margaret Striker what had happened to lead the interns and residents on 3H astray with Mr. Berman. "And none of the tests done on him beforehand had turned up much that was significant either. And then, of course, he *was* referred to us with a diagnosis of histiocytosis; that could have explained the occasional elevation in liver enzymes. . . . Well, after we'd chased that one, Richards got going on SBE and brain lesions too, and when Dr. Newman suggested taking another look at the guy's liver functions, I guess it just went by everybody. . . ."

"It was too ordinary a diagnosis for Richards," Margaret Striker cut in sharply. "He prefers fancier diseases."

"No, Margaret," Eliot Cantor responded, loyally defending his fellow intern, "Richards *is* brilliant. He really does know an awful lot of medicine. You're just down on him because he doesn't tell you nurses what he's up to some of the time. But we all messed up on Mr. Berman," he insisted, "besides—even if we had proven the hepatitis right away, the poor guy's liver was pretty well shot when we got him anyhow. . . ."

"Oh, Eliot," said Margaret Striker, grimacing, "the trouble with you is you're too nice. Admit it. Richards *is* aggressive. So is Gross-

83

man. So is Newman. All three are typical test nuts, and medicine is one great ego trip for them. If you *knew* how many times I've seen doctors order five barium enemas for some frail old lady when one was too much, you'd be stunned. Why, there isn't a nurse in this hospital who couldn't tell you horror stories about some of your more zealous colleagues!"

"Margaret," Cantor answered emphatically, "no doctor does tests for no reason! You just can't neglect any test that might tell you something you don't know about your patient because invariably, when you do, you miss the one piece of information you needed most. . . . Look at Berman," he added defensively, "that's the kind of case that gives me nightmares."

"Come on, Eliot," the head nurse replied sternly. "Isn't it sometimes just as bad to go on too long as it is to miss a diagnosis? I mean—isn't it just as important to know when to *stop* as it is to get the final answer on certain cases? I, for one, would be willing to bet that you guys do as much harm with too many tests as with too few," she continued passionately, her blue eyes flashing. "Look at what happened with poor little Mr. Bennett. If Steve Newman hadn't been on your back all the time, wouldn't you honestly have preferred just to leave him alone?"

"What are you doing Saturday?" Cantor asked, nicely sidestepping the nurse's thrust, one he recognized as containing a classic complaint many of the nurses in this hospital had against its doctors. "If it's still pleasant, do you want to drive out to Jones Beach or aren't you off?"

"I'd love to go to the beach," Margaret Striker answered, blushing slightly, glad to back off from an argument she did not much want to pursue with this intern in particular. "And please understand that I know you couldn't just quit with Mr. Bennett," she apologized, aware that she had touched a painful point with her friend. "What happened with him was something no one could have predicted," she added, "and you are definitely *not* on my list of overaggressive doctors. . . ."

Of all Newman's complement of doctors, Eliot Cantor seemed to Margaret Striker the least self-assured and hence the least as-

sertive with his patients. In many ways the chief resident's opposite, Cantor—shy, soft-spoken and easygoing—had none of the
quicksilver brilliance of Newman or Richards, and tended to be
plodding in his approach to medicine. But precisely because he
was not certain of himself, Cantor was willing to concede something that Newman and some of the other doctors found it difficult to admit: that he was afraid of his responsibility for human
life—that diagnostic enigmas terrified him and that, goaded by
his own fear of inadequacy, he ran as much risk of pushing a patient too far in his search for answers as he did of missing a diagnosis altogether. And with eighty-four-year-old Herbert Bennett,
Eliot Cantor suspected that he and everyone else had, indeed,
gone too far.

Cantor had admitted Herbert Bennett in congestive heart
failure on the same Friday night in August that Mr. Gutzman
ruptured his spleen. Nominally, the unfortunate old gentleman
had been his patient since, though almost every doctor on Newman's staff had treated him in the interim. Miraculously, that
frail little man had survived a near fatal respiratory collapse in
the wake of a nursing error with little ill effect. He had been
weaned from the MAI eight days after the accident and though
he had suffered minor brain damage that caused him afterward
to "hear angels singing," a phenomenon he visibly enjoyed, he
appeared quite normal otherwise.

As he began to recover, Dr. Cantor, Dr. Blaine, and Margaret
Striker and her nurses had worked hard for him, and by the last
week in August Mr. Bennett's condition had been dramatically improved. But on the day Mr. Bennett was pronounced ready to go
home the social worker assisting on the case learned that through
some bureaucratic error Mr. Bennett's welfare-supported apartment had been turned over to someone else during his stay in the
hospital. Another would have to be found for him—a process that
might take weeks.

On September first, Mr. Bennett had developed a urinary-tract
infection—"hospitalitis," Margaret Striker had called it, predict-

ing a chain of difficulties. "Get him out of here," Steve Newman had warned, confirming her notion, "or there'll be hell to pay."

Two days later Mr. Bennett had begun inexplicably to faint. "TIA," Dr. Richards had pronounced learnedly, arguing transient ischemic attacks—episodes of lack of oxygen to the brain caused by transient shutdowns of the tiny arteries that radiate within its surfaces.

"Electrolytes," countered Newman suggesting that the tiny particles of various salts that carry the electrical charges which govern the body's metabolism were concentrating at abnormal levels in Mr. Bennett's blood as a result of poor kidney function. The blood tests showed that Newman was right—but also that Mr. Bennett was anemic.

"Are his kidneys being properly profused?" wondered Richards, suggesting that they order a pyelography—a procedure which tests kidney function by flooding the organs with a radioactive dye and filming its movement on X-ray.

"Leave him alone," protested Cantor. "He's eighty-four. That's a risky procedure. He could be allergic to the dye and besides— even prepping him could kill him, with all those enemas. . . ."

The pyelogram was done, over Cantor's objection, without mishap; it proved nothing. Mr. Bennett began having minor convulsions.

"Liver?" questioned Newman. "CVA," countered Richards in chart rounds—cerebral vascular accidents, tiny clots thrown to the brain. They did a brain scan, also without results.

"Try a spinal tap," someone suggested.

"Don't," Cantor responded.

The tap was done and left Mr. Bennett whimpering in pain. It revealed that the potassium in the spinal fluid was as high as it was in the blood but yielded no other significant result. "Liver," Newman said again.

They did a needle biopsy. Mr. Bennett in this period lost the ability to speak. The urinary-tract infection flared. While treating this someone got careless and managed to dehydrate him. The twitching continued in his arms.

"Liver flap?" asked Dr. Blaine, looking singularly unhappy at her own suggestion.

The needle biopsy returned negative. The twitch persisted.

"CVA," growled Richards.

Cantor got the urinary-tract infection under control and Mr. Bennett's serum potassium levels began dropping. No one knew exactly why. He began to speak but couldn't remember what year it was. He suggested to Dr. Cantor, with some embarrassment, "It might be 1952?" And then confessed he'd "been hearin' angels singing most of the time now."

The first week in September Dr. Cantor sent off a final urinary-tract culture. It turned up signs of tuberculosis. He had Mr. Bennett's sputum cultured and the labs confirmed the disease on the day the social worker announced to Margaret Striker that she had obtained a new apartment and home care for Mr. Bennett. When she learned that Mr. Bennett was now classified as having an infectious disease both had to be canceled. Mr. Bennett would now have to be placed in a city hospital for infectious diseases as soon as new papers for him could be put through the bureaucratic mill.

"What kind of a hospital is it?" the head nurse had asked the social worker, a woman knowledgeable in such matters.

"Neglectsville," was her reply. "A few years ago there were three hundred patients to each RN. They've improved it now but not much. Swell—huh? It might have been better," she added, "if your guys had just skipped that last diagnosis."

Eliot Cantor, for one, wished fervently that they had. After the sputum culture returned clear evidence of active TB in Mr. Bennett's lungs Cantor had checked the standard reference on the disease to discover, to his dismay, the following notation: "'With the caseation necrosis of tuberculosis, a considerable lesion may remain solid and may become walled off by fibrous tissue; in these circumstances, no tubercle bacilli are discharged —and there is a strong tendency for the bacilli in the lesion to be sterilized. This situation may endure for months or years. Then, for reasons that are obscure and may be as diverse as long continued mental or physical fatigue . . . the bronchial communications open . . . and the conditions are ideal for multiplication of the tubercle bacilli. . . ." He had read the passage to Margaret Striker and then remarked bitterly: "Interesting, huh? That old guy fought New York's pollution, poverty, old age, and congestive heart failure, and still held off latent TB—that is, until we miracle workers set to work on him. He was tough—but he couldn't withstand us, could he?"

Chapter 15

Margaret Striker's objections to the aggressiveness of several of the doctors on 3H was not unusual. This complaint was commonplace among nurses in many major hospitals who found the practice of medicine was often less compassionate than cerebral, and the head nurse's criticism was one that pointed to the tip of a proverbial iceberg. For in many ways, Doctors Newman, Grossman, and Richards were representative of a particular breed of physician that had come to dominate American medicine in the last two decades and reordered its establishment by bringing the teaching hospitals, which had become their power bases, into pre-eminence.

Products of an era in which the class sizes in the nation's medical schools had quietly but deliberately been kept limited because of a policy of "professional birth control" advocated by the American Medical Association and other conservative groups as concerned with preventing an "overrun" of physicians in the medical marketplace as with preserving the quality of medical care, these doctor-scientists were essentially competitive scholars groomed by years of academic training to be achievers. Interested in demonstrating their prowess in specialized techniques and research, most had gravitated toward the teaching hospitals to establish themselves professionally because these institutions reflected their own special interests and were the main arenas where those who sought recognition in advanced medicine had to perform.

Bred to be winners, these scientist-physicians soon took over the various chairmanships in the teaching hospitals, and it was not long before these institutions began to resemble in spirit the men who controlled them. Biased toward research rather than patient care, the hospitals became competitive entities themselves and vied with each other for the biggest share of the bonanza in federal funds that was poured into medical "R and D" in the decade from the mid-1950s to the 1960s. Their growth in that era was swift and phenomenal and they became vast technological and research complexes. Extolled as "centers of excellence" from which all that was promising in medicine seemed to flow, the more these hospitals grew, they more they drew money, power, and talent to themselves until a scant two dozen emerged to dominate the American medical landscape like so many baronies in a feudal kingdom.

But while the great hospitals prospered, the price of their excellence was being paid in subtle ways by those never consulted about the costs—the general public. For as medicine became more complex and relied more and more heavily on expensive hardware and advanced research, two things happened: medical costs soared and the doctor patient relationship was drastically altered.

The elevating costs of hospital care had several effects. As institutional charges and doctors' fees climbed, the price of insurance to cover these costs rose rapidly and the taxes needed to pay the bills of the elderly and medically indigent went up and up and up. And though the very rich, who could command the price of superior medical service could still buy it, those with limited means found physicians hard to afford and increasingly hard to find. For as the decade of the 1970s began, the nation had a shortage of 50,000 doctors, and as the major hospitals absorbed increasing numbers of new graduates into subspecialties that made them dependent on these well-equipped centers to practice, fewer and fewer physicians were available to staff the poorer, outmoded, and often overcrowded metropolitan and small-city hospitals or to do primary care. Internists who had been expected to replace the old-time general practitioners as family doctors were in shortest supply; there was one for every 4,000 in the country in 1973 when one to every 759 was considered adequate. Even the American Medical Association, which had helped engineer the overall shortage, began to complain that these internists were poorly "distributed," and confessed that there were 134 counties in 36 states entirely without any physician and hundreds more with only one. In some western states people had to drive a hundred miles or more to see a doctor, no matter what the emergency, and even where physicians were plentiful they were concentrated in peculiar ways.

In Boston, for instance, nine out of every ten internists, obstetricians, and pediatricians served the wealthier forty per cent of the population, leaving a harried ten per cent of the doctors to take care of the collective needs of everyone else. In New York, where a similar pattern of distribution with reference to patient income existed, the needs of the poor and middle class for primary as well as acute care had been thrust on the emergency rooms, the clinics, and the general service units of public and voluntary hospitals like the one in which Margaret Striker and Eliot Cantor served.

Caught in the squeeze, these facilities soon became strained as their staffs grew smaller and their budgets became more crimped. The worst situations prevailed in the public hospitals that had accumulated no wealth of funding to begin with. In these, staffing ratios were horrendous, and it was not unusual for one registered nurse to have charge of two hundred beds at night and for a driven handful of doctors to preside over hundreds of acutely ill patients. People began to die in these institutions for lack of sufficient staff, and New York faced a crisis of deadly proportions by 1975. For though the pressures on the municipal hospitals had been eased briefly in the mid-1960s when the Health and Hospitals Corporation was set up and a program of affiliations with the city's seven teaching institutions brought an infusion of talent into them, by 1975 the public hospitals were staffed primarily by foreign doctors, some of whom barely spoke English, and, financially, they were approaching insolvency. Medically speaking, the rich were rich, but the poor grew poorer, and as costs soared and service deteriorated in the public hospitals fewer doctors opted for service in them.

The major medical centers could not, of course, take private physicians to task for the preference of the majority to work in wealthier urban and suburban neighborhoods where they would treat patients who could pay their bills. They showed similar financial predilections in patient care. Nor could they be faulted for moves they made to preserve themselves financially when confronted simultaneously with runaway costs and cutbacks in federal funding for research and Medicaid patients that had made it possible for the poor to use their more expensive facilities. Faced with too many patients seeking admission through their emergency rooms and clinics who were without insurance coverage of any sort, and burdened with the increasing costs of maintaining their own technological superiority, some began quietly and methodically cutting back on their "public service," shutting down some clinics, limiting emergency room services, and tightening the already tight budgets on the general service units like 3H, to which they now admitted only those who could pay their way, unless a patient's need was overwhelming or he or she represented interesting "teaching material" for the house staff.

The major medical centers offered no apology for this kind of selectivity. Charged with the responsibility of training physicians for the future and of maintaining their own high standards, these institutions were less concerned with general patient problems than with advancing medical science. In ordering their priorities, they chose to continue to spend on development, research, and training. But as new buildings equipped with things like linear accelerators, cobalt machines, and hyperbaric chambers went up, so did hospital fees. Costs of patient care passed an average of $250 a day on units like 3H, even though such floors were being run with half the necessary nursing staff and were short of basic supplies like sheets, pajamas, and bedpans. And while the doctors

91

in training were encouraged to pursue "excellence," and leadership in their profession continued to go to those physicians who were the most cerebral and aggressive, the quality of patient care on units like 3H was deteriorating.

Chapter 16

Though not by nature solitary, Margaret Striker lived alone by choice. Since her appointment as head nurse on 3H, interludes of silence had become essential to her. The moment at day's end when she bolted the door to her small West Side apartment and stood in the dumb peace of its four white walls, alone, was one she had come to prize. Free here of any but the demands she chose to make upon herself, the serenity of her private world on weekend days restored her. But on Sunday, when she had wakened to the sound of sea gulls mewing as they circled high above the city, she was restless. Her Saturday at the beach with Eliot Cantor had been an unqualified success and she knew, as she sat sipping her coffee in bed that morning, that she would have liked nothing better than to share the sunlight streaming through her bedroom window with him. But certain things the intern had said while they were driving cityward returned that morning to disturb her.

As Eliot Cantor had described his future plans and compared them with those of several of the other doctors on 3H, Margaret Striker had recognized that in contrast to their many professional options her own in nursing were limited. Cantor, for instance, had decided to step out of the mainstream of medicine to complete a Ph.D. the next year in preparation for a career in industrial medicine. The others, though their goals were more predictable, had chosen specializations that would offer them increasing challenge, satisfaction, and compensation as the years passed. Newman had opted for cardiology, Eaglesbury was headed into radiology, and Kate Blaine had decided to become a psychiatrist. But Margaret Striker had already reached a plateau in her own career, and beyond it there were few opportunities open to her in hospital nursing. Her diploma did not qualify her to teach professionally, and though her experience was broad and clinical competence well established, there were few positions open to her in hospital nursing in which she could utilize her talents fully. Instead, by the perverse logic of the old hierarchical system that nursing had inherited from Florence Nightingale and the Victorians, as her performance improved with experience, a nurse was usually advanced to positions that provided her with less and less opportunity to use her skills. Each step up the professional ladder took her farther from the patient's bedside so that at the head nurse's level, rather than being able to concentrate solely on directing patient care, Margaret Striker's energies were dissipated on dozens of non-nursing tasks, and those who moved up one more rung to supervisory positions not only rarely dealt with patients but were powerless even as administrators to correct the abuses of a system that kept nurses entirely subservient to doctors. This arrangement, by cancelling the incentives for growth within the profession, assured that nursing's best practitioners would be its most frustrated, and that only those who accepted the increasing fragmentation of the nursing role and eschewed all ambition to remain in the profession's lower ranks could expect to be rewarded by the knowledge that their skills were of real benefit to their patients.

As Margaret Striker sat sipping her coffee in bed that morning, gazing up at the sea gulls that swung lazily across a patch of blue framed by high-rise towers that was her piece of the sky, she could not but wonder whether nurses accepted this peculiar situation because their expectations had deliberately been kept limited by the doctors and administrators who gained from their subservience or whether, for fundamental emotional reasons, they chose to define themselves in immediate, physical terms, just as it seemed to her women had done traditionally as keepers of the hearth, the home and the young since time immemorial.

It was not, she realized, a question she could answer easily, ei-

93

ther from her knowledge of her own motivations or from those of her staff. Though most of the nurses on 3H paid lip service to feminist goals, they were not an introspective lot. Getting up and beginning to stir about in her small bedroom, Margaret Striker thought that perhaps it was because there was always too much they had to *do*, always too much muck and blood, too much final pain and too much grief to be dealt with for them to have energy left over to examine their own psychic distress or to argue with the inequities of a system that seemed quite willing to treat them shabbily. As the doctors had become increasingly preoccupied with their own pursuit of new technology and theory and with refinements in procedures, they had had less and less time to spend at the patients' bedsides, and the emotional vacuum that they had left there had quietly been filled by nurses. It was very often the nurse who held the hands of the dying in the long slow afternoons of their fear. It was she who brought comfort to the distracted families, involved herself in the nitty-gritty realities of pain, and tried to create the connections that might make life livable for the lost people in her charge. More than once Margaret Striker recalled arguing that she took little interest in the women's lib movement because it seemed to have no immediate bearing on the day-long duet of death and life which was her reality. "There is nothing to be ashamed of," she could remember protesting with no small anger when challenged with the argument that nurses enjoyed being martyrs, "in taking care of people who are desperately sick and need your skills, and I for one am proud to be able to do it." But on this quiet Sunday morning, padding about barefoot in the silence of the apartment —a silence that would normally have been soothing—Margaret Striker wondered unhappily if she still believed in her own argument. "My God, have we been conned?" she asked herself out loud, with the startled sensation of having turned over a tumbler in the lock of her own mind as she realized that the resentment she had discovered in herself might have its echo among her staff, "or have we conned ourselves?" The question focused her thoughts and she found herself recalling a conversation with her assistant head nurse, Marie Velasquez, that seemed to hold part of its answer.

Small, square-hipped, and swarthy, Marie Velasquez was the kind of person Margaret Striker admired—a woman who seemed to have an interior sense of balance the head nurse knew she herself still lacked. Married, the mother of two small children, the youngest born just a few months before Margaret Striker had taken over on the ward, Marie was some seven years older than the head nurse and a rare exception to the rule that nurses did not stay in the same job for more than a year or two; Marie had been a nurse on 3H for eight years. "Where would I go?" she would reply with a shrug when asked why she didn't move on or move up. "I'm a New York Puerto Rican, an ethnic. My people are here. They use this unit. I'm useful to them because I know how they feel, what they're afraid of. Besides, I'm not a flibberti-jibbet; I've seen enough of lives messed up to appreciate stability in my own."

When the previous head nurse had announced her decision to resign, it had been assumed by most of the 3H nursing staff that Marie's seniority guaranteed her promotion to the job even though she had been finishing up a maternity leave at the time. When Margaret Striker had been appointed head nurse instead, many of the "old hands" on 3H had held it against her even though Marie, quietly but firmly, had let it be known that she herself felt no resentment toward the new head nurse. "I wouldn't have wanted all the hassle that goes with being head nurse," she had told them. "I don't want to try to be boss to my friends and I don't want to be so worn out with responsibility that when I get home at night I've got nothing left for my kids and my husband. That's how it is," she had declared. "I put my family first because that's where my happiness and strength come from." But to Margaret Striker in private Marie had later added another reason. "I'm not sure," she had confessed, "that I can keep up with all the fancy new medicine you seem to have to know as head nurse. *Is* my practical experience enough?" she had asked. "I don't believe it could be. And I don't have time to study, you

know, *and* try to run a family *and* do a decent job every day."
Marie had made these remarks so unemotionally that Margaret
Striker had simply accepted them at face value and assumed that
whatever her disappointment about not being offered the head
nurse's job, a conflict did exist between Marie's professional and
private lives that made her unwilling to seek more responsibility
on 3H. But she wondered now if this was so. Viewed in terms of
the very real frustrations built into the head nurse's job, Marie
Velasquez's lack of professional ambition and her assistant's reluctance to fight for advancement suddenly appeared less specific
to Marie's situation as a working wife than generic to the profession as a whole.

Marie had become a nurse to care for the sick and because she
knew she would have to sacrifice her place at the bedside to advance professionally, she had chosen to accept an essentially unfair bargain in order to conserve her own usefulness as a nurse.
There was no incentive for her to scramble up to the head
nurse's position only to find her energies wasted in organizational
chores and though it did exasperate her that the anachronistic
concepts of her profession which placed nurses in the role of the
physician's handmaiden still prevailed on 3H, she was beyond
quarreling with this. She had found an affirmation of her own
humanity in nursing that made private ambition seem petty and
vain.

But there were other reasons why Marie Velasquez did
not bridle at the limits imposed upon her as a nurse quite as
much as Margaret Striker did. A conventional woman from a culture that traditionally required women to remain cloistered in
the home, Marie had managed to achieve a certain freedom and
professional independence outside her marriage without having
disrupted the equilibrium between machismo and maternity on
which it was based. By following a career in nursing and limiting
her ambitions to providing good patient care Marie was fulfilling
expectations not far different from those that applied to her as a
wife and mother. By drawing her professional and private worlds
into harmony she had used both to reinforce her own sense of

96

womanliness. For Marie this was a compromise that worked. It had freed her from tradition and allowed her to become a new kind of multipurpose woman able to live squarely in the present as a wife-mother-professional and, having achieved this kind of balance in her life, Marie was far less at cross purposes with herself, Margaret Striker now realized, than she was with her mixed ambitions and longings, or for that matter less at cross-purposes than most of the other American nurses on the ward seemed to be. Except for Marion Ping, who was also married, and Marianna Singh, whose attitudes were highly influenced by her Indian background, most of the rest of the staff on 3H seemed to be drifting uneasily between yesterday and tomorrow—wanting both to be free and independent and yet drawn irresistibly toward the goals of marriage and motherhood, which they had been raised to consider ultimately as their proper feminine purpose. Caught halfway between the conventions and expectations of the past and their own youthful uncertainties, the American nurses in particular seemed to Margaret to be incapable of forming any clear notions of what they wanted in life either as women or as professionals. Ellen King, a golden girl from the west who had tried marriage and found it wanting, despite a professed concern about women's lib was still unable to make any long-range commitment to nursing and intended one day to marry again. Sonya Craig, creamy brown and beautifully smug in her black pride and ripe womanliness, had no ambitions on 3H other than asserting her own earthy compassion and competence in promoting the interests of her less assertive black sisters. Dot Mass, thirty and frightened of it, had evidently become a nurse for one reason only, to marry a doctor, and as that possibility had become more remote, her competence had declined.

Even Melinda Kracow and Janet St. Clair, both of whom had exchanged their girlish dreams of love and marriage for more temporary liaisons, were without any particular professional aim and would, it seemed to Margaret Striker, have gladly traded their present liberated states for more traditional arrangements.

She too must feel the same ambivalence, she now realized, if a single pleasant day with Eliot Cantor could produce in its wake such a storm of contrary emotions mixing the envy she experienced when she compared her own limited hopes as a woman and a nurse to his with a wakening affection for the intern that stirred in her all the remembered longings for love, marriage, and children that she had felt in girlhood. As she considered her mixed feelings that quiet Sunday morning Margaret Striker knew that for all her struggle to free herself from home and the past, she was as much caught in the conventions that defined what was appropriate to her as a woman as any other nurse on 3H was.

Chapter 17

On Monday, Margaret Striker posted a set of assignments for the ward's nurses that gave notice to all that she intended to break up the established cliques on the floor and force those who had never assumed any kind of professional responsibility to take it. Melinda Kracow, an LPN, was to train for team leadership so she could run one side of the ward when necessary, and Janet St. Clair was to be moved up to "charge" nurse on occasion, taking responsibility for many of the head nurse's duties on days when Margaret Striker or Marie Velasquez was too busy. But her surprised staff had barely digested this realignment when Dr. Newman appeared at the nursing station to announce a series of discharges and admissions and give Margaret Striker a brief but disturbing report.

"I'm sending home three this morning and taking in two electives this afternoon and an ER admission. One's a Hodgkin's for staging, one's probable AML, and would you believe it, one's just a rule-out MI."

"How many are male and how many female, or am I to run a coeducational room?" the nurse asked good-humoredly. "And, if you don't mind, Doctor, do they have names?"

"The Hodgkin's is a girl named Mary O'Malley, twenty-six. The

98

AML is a lady just diagnosed as leukemic here in clinic last Thursday. They think she's an acute myelogenous and not monocytic and she's probably got some chance for remission. I think she's signed an informed consent to be treated under the protocols. Her name is Olsen, Tanya Olsen. And I'm sending home two hearts, Fink and Byrne, both nicely adjusted on 'dig,' and that old lady with angina in 316 who never shoulda been admitted here in the first place, Mrs. Twining. Oh yeah, the MI is a lady named Suarez. And then we're second up for another admission through the ER, I'm told, so I'll have to start borrowing beds." He did a small shuffle step, turned around once, lightly, and grinned at the head nurse sassily.

"I take it from the action that you were on over the weekend, Dr. Newman?" the nurse remarked, glancing at her chart rack momentarily to sort out which patients coming in that morning would go where. "And I heard some new names at report—so would you mind telling me about those admissions too?"

"I take it from the sunburn you were at the beach this weekend, Miss Striker," Newman responded mischievously. "And, as only one of my interns is also sunburned, I must conclude that there was fraternizing going on. You know I don't approve of that. However. To business. Yes, I was on, and yes, I do have a couple of more things to tell you. On Mr. Blumenthal, our resident hemophiliac, we haven't been able to stop the bleed this time so we're going to have to start pushing up the factor eight. So pray, do novenas, light candles, or whatever suits you. And Mrs. Toranado? I guess you heard we lost her on Sunday. Must have been fungal, by the way. The Gentomycin didn't touch the fever. Bad scene. The husband was in there when she went out. But it was subdural, not sepsis. He went completely nuts and had to be carried away and tranquilized. Jesus. Messy. She went so fast, you know. I mean, diagnosed three weeks ago, expired Sunday. Thirty-three. Two kids. Not nice . . ." He paused, drumming his fingers on the desk in front of him, distracted momentarily.

"What happened, Steve, no platelets?"

"Yeah, no platelets at all Sunday. But what the hell, Margaret, you know it wasn't really a matter of platelets. She turned out to be a promelocytic leukemia—no chance at all." His voice trailed off. He continued to drum his fingers on the desk, his shiny gold wedding band tapping a tattoo on the formica surface.

"Is there something else I should know about besides the admissions, Dr. Newman?" Margaret Striker asked softly, certain now that the normally irrepressible chief resident was holding something back and that, after all, Eliot Cantor's favorable estimate of Newman might be correct.

"I mean, the other new admissions aren't all infectious diseases requiring isolation, are they?"

He grinned momentarily and shook his head. "No," he said, "I replaced Mrs. Toranado with a nice quiet old lady with advanced arterial sclerosis in congestive heart failure Sunday night. She thinks she's the Duchess of Windsor and that I'm the Duke, even though I'm not the right shape. So when you go into 322 just tell her the duke sent and she'll be cooperative. The other guy, though, *is* a little difficult. He's a lawyer with reticulum cell sarcoma. He was supposed to be in remission last spring after they treated him here. He might be in diabetic trouble now or he might have an occult infection since he's been on prednisone, and it might also be almost anything else 'cause he's got a lot of goofy symptoms. Anyway, I've set him up with a diet to do a glucose tolerance test and the cultures today may get us somewhere too. No, it's not the Sunday admissions. It's Jane Day. There are new orders on Jane. You'll see 'em." He dropped his voice slightly. "How long has she been here, Margaret, do you know offhand?"

"I'll check," the head nurse responded quietly, reaching for Jane Day's chart. "Here it is. She was admitted on June twenty-eighth through the ER and was listed then as an FUO."

When admitted in June, Jane Day, a diabetic with a severely enlarged heart, had come to 3H from the emergency room with a high fever of unknown origin that was peaking at 105°. Within two days of her arrival she had apparently suffered a series of small strokes that had partially paralyzed her on the left side, so that after the doctors had controlled both her diabetes, exacerbated by her high fever, and the infection that had been causing the fever, it had been necessary to keep her on the ward until institutional placement under Medicaid became available. During the last week in July, while she was waiting for placement in a nursing home, Jane Day had lost the ability to swallow—evidently the result of still another small "cerebral vascular accident," as the strokes she had been experiencing had been labeled. After that it had been necessary for the nurses to feed her through a naso-gastric tube and she had declined steadily and slowly, so that by mid-August she was only partially conscious. On August twenty-fifth her lungs had begun to fill with fluids, threatening congestive heart failure. Margaret Striker had given the nurses directions to suction her lungs but eventually, when they could no longer fight the choking collection of fluids, the doctors "trached" her and put her on a respirator. During that week, whenever the doctors searched for new veins that could withstand intravenous implants she had moaned and on several occasions superficial surgical procedures which exposed veins below the surface were required to continue therapy. On September first, after seven days on the respirator, she was weaned from it successfully but did not regain consciousness. She was given sustenance by tube feedings, IV ampicillin to control infection, and insulin as required to control her diabetes, but the nurses had not been able to check the development of open ulcers along her spine.

"What's with her now, Steve?" the nurse asked, looking up from her rapid review of Jane Day's bleak record. "What more can we add to this mess?"

"Nothing," Newman answered in a curiously flat voice. "She's been throwing multiple emboli to her brain over the past week; I'm sure of it."

"And?"

"And—like I said—they've written some new orders on her. Poor old girl." He pursed his lips and without further comment turned smartly and hustled down the hall, his gait slightly rolling. "Make rounds with us if you can this morning—there may be some interesting stuff developing . . ." he called over his shoulder to the startled head nurse, who had watched him with a sense of revelation as he walked away.

"I'll try," she responded, aware now that Dr. Newman wanted her approval this morning. "And thank you . . ." It saddened Margaret Striker when she checked her books to find, as she had surmised from Newman's remarks, that Jane Day's orders for ampicillin had been reduced by one half. But the move was one she approved in human terms despite its professional significance. For by reducing the antibiotic that had for so long protected the unconscious woman from infection the doctors were opening the way for nature to take a course they had heretofore blocked. Though the decision in no way represented "mercy killing"—for no one was acting overtly to end Jane Day's life and all the other measures supporting her existence and comfort would continue—it was evident, nevertheless, that over the weekend the doctors had made up their minds to step back a little from the battle with death in room 326.

"No code 700 on Jane," Margaret Striker mumbled to Marie Velasquez, who had joined her at the nursing station and who responded with only a slight lift of one eyebrow. "And I'm going to go on rounds with the doctors this morning to get caught up. Newman asked me and I think I should."

"Do as your chief commands," Marie responded lightly. "No 700 huh? Sensible. Newman's idea?"

"Indirectly—yes," said the head nurse. "And he also has elected to discharge three this morning and admit three more this afternoon," she told her assistant. "But let's let the nursing assignments hold as they are because after rounds I'm still hoping to start orienting Melinda and Janet. I want Melinda to move up to team leading and Janet to be able to take charge by October. The others are going to gripe, especially Obakwanga, because I know I won't be able to push Melinda too fast. But I think it's time those two took on more challenge and shaking the place up will be good for the gripers, too—give 'em something to think about anyway. What do you think?"

"Whew," Marie Velasquez responded easily. "You're all energy today. But I guess we are due for a shape-up around here—and two more chiefs among the Indians sounds useful to me."

The first portion of rounds that morning were at the bedside and Margaret Striker followed the doctors through the ward, feeling awkward with Eliot Cantor in Newman's presence. She concentrated her attention so strictly on the rapidfire analysis of each patient's problems that until the group turned into the room where Harold Blumenthal sat crouched in his wheelchair like some shy, subterranean animal, she had given no further thought to how he might react to Newman's announcement that he finally had become refractory to conventional treatment for hemophilia.

"Does it take all of you to stop one little ulcer from bleeding," he asked, smiling wanly up at the semicircle of doctors grouped around him, his pale skin drawn sharply over his peaked nose but hanging loosely at the jawline like an ill-fitting garment. "Or is that why you brought Miss Striker along—because she and her girls have done such wonders for me in the past?"

"We've got some difficult news for you, Mr. Blumenthal," Newman responded, shoving his hands into his trouser pockets and looking directly into Blumenthal's tobacco-colored eyes. "We're going to have to go for broke this time and push up your concentrate."

"It's that bad?" asked Blumenthal, almost philosophically. "You can't stop the bleeding otherwise?"

"You know how it works," Newman answered honestly. "You're as much of an expert on your disease as any of us. No, we haven't succeeded in stopping this bleed, so you'll be getting more blood today to help out. But you've developed a resistance to the concentrated factor eight in lower quantities so we've got to try to bomb out the antibodies and the circulating anticoagulants you've developed that are destroying the effectiveness of the AHF you've been getting. Then we ought to get a percentage gain that'll let you start clotting again and stop this bleeding. . . ."

Mr. Blumenthal, pensive but impassive, held Newman's look for a moment and then let his head drop forward slightly, like a man offering his neck to the guillotine, acknowledging with this single nod that he understood perfectly what the chief resident had just told him.

There was little, in fact, that Harold Blumenthal and his wife, Darlene Ryan Blumenthal, did *not* know about the mechanics and treatment of hemophilia or about his prognosis. Blumenthal had lived with his dangerous inherited defect of the blood's ability to clot for more than sixty years and from the stories he and his wife had recounted to Margaret Striker over the two years she had known them, his disease had become the central factor in both of their lives.

"When I was a kid," Blumenthal had told the head nurse, "all you could do was lie in a corner and hope you wouldn't die. . . . Some of us went crazy that way, I know. But I survived. And in time I learned to live."

Unable to go to school in the years before there was any effective treatment for hemophilia, Blumenthal had grown up as if he lived in a bell jar, a recluse from the world and yet an avid observer of all that transpired beyond his reach. Taught by his mother to read, he had participated in life at a distance through newspapers and radio. During the years of World War II the places in the news became the terrain of his imagination and the faces that began to emerge from the holocaust became his companions in loneliness; he remembered Colin Kelly and Roger Young; he remembered Lidice; he remembered the photographs from Dachau at war's end. "I began to realize then," he once told Margaret Striker, "that *every* life is hazardous and that in all those years of prayer and anguish I'd been misusing the only one I had. . . ."

In the years just after the war Harold Blumenthal, then in his early thirties, met Darlene Ryan. A squat woman with the luminous eyes and determined expression of her Irish forebears, she was a receptionist and records' keeper at the office of a doctor to whom Blumenthal had been referred when he developed one of the common complications of his disease, crippling hemarthritis, in both knees as a result of repeated hemorrhaging into the

104

joints. A generous, motherly person with a broad streak of Irish romanticism in her soul, Darlene Ryan's sympathetic nature had often involved her in other people's troubles, and in Harold Blumenthal, now alone in the world after his mother's death, she saw not only a brave and lonely man who needed help but a suffering human being whose cause wanted championing. It was not long before they were partners in a marriage, which, though curious, proved a happy one nevertheless.

As a professional Margaret Striker knew that people who must live with the very real possibility that each day could be the last for them could become incredibly dodgy with their emotions and she had often seen people erect intricate psychological defenses, alone or in pairs, that could distort any relationship. Some developed elaborate charades of denial that tied them together in a web of guilt and fear which could erupt in misplaced rage. Others drew together in a kind of exaggerated mutuality which formed a fortress against terror that permitted both to appear brave, until the fortress fell. And it seemed to the head nurse that the latter had been the case with Darlene and Harold Blumenthal.

"Before I met and married Darlene," Blumenthal had confided to Margaret Striker quite recently, "I think I'd been trying to make a deal with God, asking very very little of life so that by not appearing greedy I might convince Him to let me go on living. But Darlene was a fighter and she saw things another way. She told me, God wanted workers, not cowards, so I guess with her help I started trying to make a new deal with Him."

The defense they constructed together against his vulnerability had taken the form of an offensive against hemophilia; both became crusading activists in a then newly formed organization of hemophiliacs who were banding together to attack their problems medically, financially, and socially in mutual action. United in their cause, the Blumenthals traveled throughout New Jersey and southern New York on weekends; helping to organize blood drives, gathering funds, organizing local groups of hemophiliacs into mutual-aid societies, and trying to educate the public to the realities of this disease. On weekdays both worked—she as an accountant, he at home assembling mechanical pencils to keep up with the costs of his illness, then running about two thousand dollars a year.

"It was a strange but happy time," Blumenthal recalled in one conversation with the head nurse, "because, though I had a couple of serious bleeds in my knee and nearly lost my leg, I was discovering that the more we got out in the world, the more we both got involved with other hemophiliacs, the less time I had to worry about myself or anything else. Before I met Darlene I used to brood about things in the news a lot, but do you know what 1963 meant to me? Not Kennedy's assassination, though we both were stunned by it, but that we got Cryo. We got Cryo in 1963, and it set us free!"

Isolated from thawing frozen blood plasma, the precipitate "Cryo," as it came to be known to its users, was a concentrated form of the antihemophiliac factor labeled AHF that was present in normal blood. One of the practical achievements of the research efforts of the 1960s, it revolutionized the treatment of hemophilia. In situations of hemorrhage, where before its discovery the only treatment was to give hemophiliacs massive transfusions of plasma that posed a threat of circulatory overload and congestive heart failure, "Cryo" was effective in small quantities to stop bleeding and could also be used prophylactically to give born "bleeders" protection against their inherited defect.

"Children could go to school. They could play with other kids," Blumenthal was fond of saying, his brown eyes shining. "Young people didn't have to become cripples, like me; Cryo gave us hope —something we'd never really had before—and it gave me years with Darlene I'd probably never have enjoyed!"

But by 1972, when Margaret Striker had first met the Blumenthals, they had entered a new arena in his struggle for life. Users of Cryo or the unfrozen concentrate of AHF developed soon after its discovery could become resistant to it in time as their bodies reacted to the foreign blood factor by developing antibodies against it. Circulating in the bloodstream, these eventually acted as an anticoagulant that virtually immunized the individual against AHF and destroyed its effectiveness. After ten years of relative freedom from bleeding, Harold Blumenthal had reached this impasse. Recurrent bouts of hemorrhaging from an ulcer had brought him to the hospital over and over again in the past two years, and as his requirement for AHF increased, his resistance to it had also mounted until he had become all but refractory to treatment. Though both husband and wife affected stoicism in the face of his hazardous situation, Margaret Striker, who knew them well, having cared for Harold Blumenthal repeatedly over the past twenty-four months, was unconvinced that his cheerfulness could be accepted at face value. The dark ring of stain on his fingers marked him as a chain smoker, and his ulcer gave further mute testimony that Blumenthal was a man feeling stress.

"I'm really worried about him," she whispered to Eliot Cantor as they trailed Newman down the hall after leaving Blumenthal's room. "He seems to be just hanging on now, almost on the verge of giving in. If things go badly and he starts to fall apart, I'm afraid she may fall apart too."

"I just don't know, Margaret," Cantor replied. "You know the Blumenthals better than I ever will, and you've been around a lot more patients facing up to this kind of a tough, chancy situation than I have. But one thing I do know, Margaret, people have absolutely amazing resources.

"My God—did you know that Mrs. Toranado asked Eaglesbury when she could go home on Sunday morning? How's that for denial? And that lady, the Duchess of Windsor? Can you think of a better way to handle being old, alone, and frightened than by becoming a famous person like the duchess? Yeah—and one of these new admissions, the lawyer? Well, Steve said he was diagnosed here as sarcoma late last year—and *told* the diagnosis. Do you know what he insists is wrong with him now? Malaria. Crazy —huh? Malaria!"

Chapter 18

In one of the last rooms the doctors and head nurse visited they found Dela Hanze sitting up in her bed, quietly gabbling to herself, but at the sudden unexplained appearance of so many strangers in white she became terrified and began to howl. Just as rounds had been starting, Dr. Newman had surprised Margaret Striker by telling her that he hoped to discharge Mrs. Hanze in about a week. Though the chief resident was plainly dismayed by the woman's agitated outburst, he reiterated his intention to discharge her the moment he had completed his review of her case with the interns.

Two weeks before, when Dela Hanze, a big, strong-faced woman who looked rather like George Washington, had first been brought to 3H close to death in acidotic shock, she had shown an amazing stamina for her eighty years and made a remarkable recovery. But in the last ten days the "miracle" Dr. Newman, Dr. Blaine, and the head nurse had managed to work for her had come to seem of doubtful value. For as Mrs. Hanze had been nursed back to consciousness it had become evident that she was mentally deranged. The doctors attributed her delirium partly to the destructive effects of a chronic kidney condition on her brain, but they had also determined that Mrs. Hanze, somewhere along the line, had been addicted to Thorazine. Caught in a strange nether world of hallucination and delirium from which it now seemed there was little hope she could be returned, Mrs. Hanze seemed to spend most of her hours either trying to cope with imaginary terrors or dreaming in a Thorazine-induced stupor. Since there was little more the doctors on 3H could hope to accomplish for her medically, Steve Newman, under pressure from the hospital administration not to let chronic patients like Mrs. Hanze languish in beds needed for the acutely ill, had decided, despite her continuing derangement, that he had to discharge her.

He had therefore instructed Margaret Striker to set the bureaucratic machinery in motion to find Mrs. Hanze suitable custodial placement.

Newman's request was perfectly routine. Nominally, the doctors were still expected to request that arrangements be made for patients, like Dela Hanze, in need of special supervision on discharge. But in practice the responsibility for filing the proper papers and seeking the best available placements for them had long ago fallen to the head nurses and social workers on the wards. In any given week Margaret Striker was engaged in several complicated negotiations with the floor's case worker simultaneously as the two tried to weave together workable connections for otherwise unstrung lives, like Dela Hanze's. Therefore, she attached no particular importance to the call she placed just after rounds that morning until she began reading Mrs. Hanze's chart aloud to the social worker and realized that the story it told could only have an ugly ending unless a way could be found to circumvent the indifferent system that would soon swallow Dela Hanze's life.

In clipped medical jargon, the chart history reiterated a tale already too familiar to the head nurse, a story of neglect that summarized the way countless old people like Dela Hanze were regularly victimized by the unscrupulous who had found a way to profit from their infirmity and society's disregard for them, which in this version became the more disturbing because of certain facts about Mrs. Hanze's past.

Her chart record was not particularly thick. It began with what had been Mrs. Hanze's first hospital admission in ten years the previous May, when an insidious urinary-tract infection had flared into an acute kidney problem and noted that until just before her referral to this hospital in serious condition, Dela Hanze had been competently caring for herself and several other elderly women friends in her large West Side apartment. But the admitting resident's notes from May also contained other indicators that Dela Hanze was made of stout stuff. Included in his workup was a conventionally graphed family tree showing Mrs. Hanze's mother and father's name and suspended from theirs a line indicating that she had been one of five siblings. Slashed across every name but Mrs. Hanze's, indicating that all but she were dead, was the single word "Hitler." Reading this, Margaret Striker understood with a chill the faint line of numbers she had noticed tattooed on Dela Hanze's forearm when she had bathed her.

But the evidence of Mrs. Hanze's formidable will to live did not end with the notation that she had somehow withstood the depredations of Treblinka to arrive as the only survivor of her family in America in 1948; it was there as well in the strictly medical notes on her stay in the hospital the previous spring, when she had weathered both renal shutdown and heart failure without any noticeable impairment in her mental faculties. But in June, when it had come time for her to be discharged, Dela Hanze's luck had evidently run out at last; she had fallen afoul of what the case worker talking to Margaret Striker on the telephone described as "the great geriatrics lottery"—a lottery in lives that to the head nurse seemed suddenly to give a pathetic human focus to all the arguments against elitism in medicine Margaret Striker had read and heard about as a nurse.

The result of a great folly of mismanagement that had seen the government spending billions of dollars on medical research in efforts which had resulted in the prolongation of life without any organized provision being made to see that those science "saved" could be provided for humanely when they became incapable of looking after themselves, the "lottery," as the case worker called it, was the nonsystem that had evolved as the numbers of chronically ill, senile, and incapacitated in the United States had begun to outrun the facilities for their care, creating a scarcity of beds in nursing homes that had resulted in old people being forced to accept placement wherever it could be found. Nine times out of ten it was in privately owned institutions where, despite uniformly high costs, the standards of care were scandalously spotty and ill enforced.

When Dela Hanze had been discharged in June a nephew had placed her in a facility which, though purportedly able to provide skilled nursing care and medical supervision at somewhat less than the average $225 a week charged by several homes the hospital had recommended, had nevertheless been neither staffed nor equipped to provide Mrs. Hanze with the kind of care she had required, nor was it visited regularly by the physician who owned it. And there, if her condition on her admission to 3H could be taken as evidence, the unfortunate Mrs. Hanze had been consistently mismanaged medically and finally slugged into a stupor by the ill-considered administration of Thorazine until the combined insults of neglect and drugging had driven her first into Thorazine addiction and finally into the acidotic shock that had so nearly taken her life. Now helpless, bewildered, and chronically ill, she needed permanent custodial care and comprehensive medical supervision for what was left of her life. But to worsen a grim plight, as Margaret Striker totaled up the figures in Mrs. Hanze's chart, she found to her dismay that Mrs. Hanze had all but exhausted her Medicare benefits. Twenty days after her discharge, her family would become entirely responsible for the costs of her care in a nursing home until her life savings were exhausted and she could be declared a "medical indigent" eligible for Medicaid. Under these circumstances, it did not seem likely to Margaret Striker that her nephew could be persuaded to seek more expensive care for Mrs. Hanze or that any home other than the one where she had been placed would be willing to take her in unless her family guaranteed payment for her care for at least a month in advance, a sum in excess of one thousand dollars.

"She's pulled an awful set of numbers in the geriatrics lottery," the social worker told Margaret Striker unhappily as the nurse completed her depressing brief. "But if you can manage to stall the discharge I'll try to persuade her nephew not to send her back to that charnel house until I've made a plea for her admission to one of the better Jewish homes. Can you hold Newman off for about two weeks, anyway? Maybe I can work something for her in that space of time, but a week is absolutely impossible."

"I doubt it," Margaret Striker responded. "The pressure's on the chief resident to keep the chronic patients from ending up 'disposition cases' on the wards, so they do try to move 'em out as fast as they can to any placement you give us. But I'll try to persuade Newman to keep her on for a little bit if you think you can make a switch for her. I've decided he's not such a bad sort after all, and since she hasn't used up all her in-hospital Medicare yet, maybe if I can tell him you're onto something he'll extend her a little up here. But don't forget, Newman's leaving 3H in two weeks himself, and I've no idea who they'll send up here next. So work your shuffle before the first of October, okay? Good luck," she concluded, "and thanks."

She put down the phone, glanced at her watch, realized that she was already three minutes late for the meeting she had scheduled with Janet St. Clair and Melinda Kracow, and with a fierce gesture jammed Mrs. Hanze's chart record back onto the rack that stood against the wall behind the nursing station. Then the head nurse deliberately put the old woman's griefs out of her mind and hurried down the corridor toward her small office, her wooden clogs beating a determined rhythm as she turned her mind to the next task on her morning's checklist: teaching the two nurses she was planning to advance to "charge" how to anticipate the doctors' and patients' needs and how to order in advance, from lists of more than a thousand items from drugs to catheter tips regularly stocked by the hospital, those six or eight hundred that each week needed replenishment on 3H.

Chapter 19

"Please make me laugh!" Margaret Striker said glumly to Eliot Cantor, putting a tray down opposite him at lunch after the intern had beckoned her to his table. "I've had a terrible morning. . . ."

"Negative Q sign," said Cantor, rolling back his eyes and protruding his tongue from the left side of his opened mouth to form the shape of a reverse-tailed Q. "It means the patient has expired.

Positive Q sign." He demonstrated again, this time sticking his tongue out to the right. "Same thing; the patient is dead."

"And that's funny?" the head nurse asked, chuckling at the intern's foolishness.

"Would you rather hear about the guy who came into the ER yesterday with a blood sugar of 1,100?"

"Did he go into diabetic coma?"

"Would you believe they sent him home after giving him Orinase?"

"And that's funny?" she asked, horrified. "I don't even understand it!"

"Would you rather hear about what happened to Richards on his way to grand rounds today?"

"Does it begin, 'A funny thing happened on the way to grand rounds'?"

"No."

"Is it funny?"

"He doesn't think so, but I do."

"Then tell me what happened to Richards on the way to grand rounds."

"He met a guy in the elevator who told him he was God and the Devil. And then the guy pushed the stop button and started bouncing Richards around in there like a basketball."

"Good Lord. What happened?"

"Richards managed to push the nine and the elevator went up to psychiatric. They were standing there when the elevator doors opened."

"Who was?"

"Two security guards and two psychiatrists with a straitjacket who were out looking for God and the Devil. Do you think he was schizophrenic?"

"Oh, Eliot," said the nurse, shaking her head at her friend but laughing. "You are an idiot. How is Richards?"

"He looks like he had a Spalding in his mouth on the left side. Positive Q sign?"

"Did they really send someone who came in with the blood sugar of 1,100 home on Orinase?" she asked, ignoring the intern's mad-faced antics. "And what were you doing in the ER today anyway? We're up to our ears in electives this afternoon. Four admissions coming in after lunch and the beds they're going into are barely cool. I hope Newman isn't serious about borrowing beds for ER admissions, is he?"

"No—but only 'cause suddenly the place is nearly a full house and there aren't beds to borrow. No—the reason I was in the ER this morning is that I'm going there next month on my first month of electives."

"Oh, Eliot, I'm sorry," Margaret Striker sympathized, acknowledging that the month in the emergency room was among the most hectic in the year of an intern's training. "But I suppose you might as well get it over with."

"Don't be sorry, Margaret," Eliot Cantor replied, grinning now and reaching across the table to pat her hand. "I'll just need more tender loving care than ever next month, and you're elected." Seeing her blush, he busied himself with his sandwich before reporting with a perfectly serious face, "Yes, they did send a guy home on Orinase who came in with a blood sugar of 1,100. I couldn't believe it."

"But when the resident found out, didn't he call him back? I mean, he *could* go into a coma anyplace, couldn't he?"

"They were taking bets afterward on whether he even made it to the subway. No, they didn't call him, but he came back today on his own, still on the verge of collapsing into coma, and *this* time they admitted him."

"Eliot," she said, shaking her head at him, "that was *not* funny. That was insane."

"Yeah, well, I found it reassuring in a way. It made me realize there are actually interns around here that know *less* than I do. Now don't *you* find that somehow comforting?"

"You're hopeless, Eliot Cantor," she answered him, laughing. "Absolutely hopeless."

It was as well the lunch with Eliot Cantor restored Margaret

Striker to a more cheerful frame of mind, for when she got back to 3H just before two o'clock it had taken on the quality of macabre carnival. At the nursing station eleven doctors, including the chief resident, were all talking at once. But above the noise the head nurse could hear both phones shrilling, unattended, within their easy reach. As she raced to answer them a series of tableaux presented themselves through the doorways to the patients' rooms that heightened the impression of the ward's madness. In the room with Mr. Blumenthal she glimpsed the obese figure of a man who looked more like a stranded whale than a human lying in the bed that till this morning had been Mr. Burns's, roaring obscenities to the ceiling at the top of his voice. In the next, a two-bed room for women, another man, in scarlet pajamas, appeared to be dancing in the lilac gloom with a large bouquet of flowers. Opposite the nursing station, Mrs. Hanze, whom the head nurse had promised the social worker that morning would soon be "ambulatory in a wheelchair" to make the old woman eligible for certain nursing homes that excluded the bedridden, sat tied up in a sitting position on a large blue commode, honking, while at the end of the hallway Marie Velasquez and Mary Obak-wanga appeared close to blows as they gesticulated violently at each other. And just as the head nurse reached the nursing station Melinda Kracow emerged from a closet, impassively pushing a mop bucket before her at the same moment that Janet St. Clair appeared from the medications room, red-eyed and puffy-faced from crying, carrying the two o'clock tray of pills and potions.

The phones, of course, stopped ringing just as Margaret Striker reached them. But the din continued unabated and as she stood surveying the crowd of arguing doctors, an expression of disapproval on her face meant to quell them to silence, she saw the woman coming down the ward's corridor, carrying a battered red canvas bag bearing the legend "Tempus, Viva, et Disportati Illustrati."

She was small, not more than five feet tall, her chestnut hair and heart-shaped face unremarkable. But there was something in the lurching, hunch-shouldered walk and pallid eyes that caught

115

the nurse off guard and made her stomach turn. For as their eyes locked the stranger gave Margaret Striker a look that while distraught, almost wild, was yet so penetrating that it seemed somehow as if it had unlocked forgotten closets and cupboards in the nurse's own mind and left the doors banging and swinging irrationally as in a dream. And in that moment Margaret Striker knew with perfect clarity that the woman had not only captured her own face absolutely, registering it, the arguing doctors, Mrs. Hanze, and the sterile craziness of the ward in her mind's eye with the same uncomprehending fidelity with which a photographic plate registers light, but that in that same fraction of time she had given herself up to the mad scene, almost swooning into it like someone jumping from a bridge, surrendering her life to the indifferent doctors and the watchful nurse with an unprotesting sense of her own powerlessness.

Her name was Tanya Olsen and she had learned on Thursday at the hospital clinic that she had leukemia. The doctors had given her the probable name of her disease—acute myelocytic leukemia. They had also explained that remission from her form of cancer was sometimes obtained by patients who submitted to intensive combination chemotherapy, which involved the intentional poisoning of the affected bone marrow in hopes that healthy tissue could be induced to replace the cancerous cells wiped out by this high-risk course of treatment. But though she had signed the consent required for patients who accepted the dangerous and still experimental treatments that were the only effective ones known for leukemia and had obediently delivered herself at the appointed time to 3H, it was to become evident to Margaret Striker, who had recognized a peculiar empathy with this slight, frightened woman from the instant their eyes had met, that Tanya Olsen had, since the moment the doctors had pronounced the word "leukemia" on Thursday, been operating in a kind of trance. Unable to comprehend the stealthy treachery of the enemy that had overtaken her as she had moved unaware through her ordered days in the library where she worked, she had felt strangely betrayed. And as she had tidied up her affairs without telling her daughter or friends anything except that she was to be hospitalized for "certain tests—blood tests—that sort of thing," it had seemed to her that her body, once familiar and reliable, had been taken over by a force beyond her control. This force filled her with a wretched sense of her own helplessness and at the same time made her keenly conscious of the profligate richness of life sweeping around her like a river around a stone.

She had brought with her in the red canvas bag a toothbrush, a hairbrush, a prayer book, a pair of aqua slippers, and a sweater—but no bathrobe, no nightgown, and no change of clothes. As Margaret Striker put away the few things in room 316 she had the impression that in packing to come to 3H Tanya Olsen had refused to think about either staying in the hospital or leaving it, ever. When the nurse offered her a hospital gown she had refused it as if by accepting the anonymous white coat her identity would somehow be dissolved and she would become a part of the ward, cut off forever from the world beyond the hospital. But later that afternoon, when the head nurse stopped by to see if an aide sent to purchase her a proper nightgown had returned, Tanya Olsen seemed to be trying to come to terms with the truth of her situation. "I know what will happen," she said in a whisper as she lay motionless on her bed like some slight medieval bronze, her arms folded across her chest, her aquamarine eyes fixed on the ceiling. "I saw the movie *Love Story*. I know how it will end."

Chapter 20

Preoccupied, Margaret Striker did not react immediately to Tanya Olsen's words. Instead, they settled on the surface of her mind like a leaf on water—part of an aimless pattern of impressions that would not emerge from this day's confusions until almost two weeks later, when she would recall their poignancy. But in the rush of the moment, though the head nurse sympathized with Tanya Olsen, other concerns took precedence.

She was puzzled about what troubled Janet St. Clair, whom she was sure had been crying when she had seen her just after lunch, and she had not yet found time to see the other new female admission, the girl in for staging of her newly diagnosed Hodgkin's disease, who had come in while Margaret had been off the floor. But most pressing were the explosive issues that had suddenly been raised as a result of a scene between one of her nurses and Walter Forsyth, a newly admitted patient, which had the potential of igniting a racial quarrel within her staff and brought her own authority as head nurse into question.

The precipitating incident had occurred between one and two o'clock, while Margaret Striker had been off the floor, having lunch, when Forsyth had first been sent up to 3H. An immense man with a flowing old-testament beard and unkempt silver hair, Forsyth, had been irascible from the moment he arrived on the unit—demanding service, dissatisfied with having been put in a two-bed room, and loudly critical of everyone who tried to cope with his complaints, particularly of Mary Obakwanga, the nurse who had the misfortune to be assigned to the room in which he was lodged with Harold Blumenthal, the hemophiliac.

"The service around here is terrible," Forsyth had shouted at the nurse as soon as she had come into his room in response to his call bell. "I'm a sick man, weak. I need a bed pan. I rang and nobody came. I'm paying for service and what I get is a lazy black bitch. . . ." He had begun gesticulating wildly, his eyes distended, his face glazed with a film of sweat, and then launched into a string of obscenities laced heavily with racial slurs.

Icily polite, the African nurse had tendered him the bed pan, stood his ranting in silence for a moment, and then stalked out of the room. When she finally returned to Forsyth's bedside nearly an hour later, having ignored repeated summonses in the interim, the enraged man had thrown the bed pan at her, scattering the contents across the floor, and there had been a loud scene between them.

It was in the aftermath of this blowup that Margaret Striker had returned to the ward to see Marie Velasquez and Mary Obakwanga evidently quarreling at the end of the corridor as Melinda Kracow headed toward Forsyth's room to clean up the mess. But when the head nurse, on learning what had happened, tried to intercede, offering to relieve the Rwandan nurse of responsibility for the combative Mr. Forsyth, so long as she apologized to him, Mary Obakwanga had turned to her in a rage that went beyond the immediate trouble. She had refused to apologize to Forsyth even when the head nurse made it an order, accusing her of racism and creating a situation in which Margaret Striker now was either going to be forced to cite her officially for insubordination or to back down in what threatened to become a confrontation between herself and the more militant blacks on her staff.

Margaret Striker had long recognized the potential for this kind of racial conflict in her relationship with Mary Obakwanga. Though superficially polite, there had often been a cutting edge in Nurse Obakwanga's remarks and a certain haughtiness had long been evident in her attitude toward the head nurse's authority that Margaret Striker only partly understood. Some of the friction between them, she knew, had grown out of Mary Obakwanga's disappointment in not being promoted to the position of assistant head nurse at the time of the change in command on 3H, when it had been expected that Marie Velasquez would be advanced to the head nurse's position. The African nurse had badly wanted that promotion and when it did not come she construed Margaret Striker's appointment as racially unfair both to Marie Velasquez and to herself.

Raised in Rwanda in the early years of Uhuru, Mary Obakwanga was racially touchy and her resentment of whites went bone deep. Even though she had trained in Great Britain she had never lost her suspicion of white society and lived in a permanent state of indignation with its real and imagined inequities to blacks, a warrior easily incensed to battle, carrying her black pride like a banner.

On 3H, this militancy had quietly elevated her to a position of leadership among those to whom all things African were axiomatically admirable. Even before Margaret Striker had come to the ward Mary Obakwanga had been regarded as a spokeswoman for its racial militants and from the outset the head nurse had recognized that she represented a threat to her own authority. Aware that black pride alloyed with professional pride made for better nursing on a unit like this, the head nurse had studiously avoided any clash with Mary Obakwanga or the other militants. Mary Obakwanga and Sonya Craig were, in fact, among her most competent nurses precisely because they cared about demonstrating their own professional superiority and because, like Marie Velasquez, they had chosen to remain on this most rugged service in the belief that here they could expect to do more for their own people than on semiprivate duty. Though they did exhibit a particular sensitivity to the griefs of those patients who came to 3H bearing not only the marks of their diseases but of the depredations of the city's rotting streets, who, for the most part, were not white, they were generally even-handed in their treatment of the floor's patients and as considerate of stricken old ladies like Dela Hanze as they were of unfortunates like Herbert Bennett and Jane Day, so that Margaret Striker had only found more to praise in their devotion than to quarrel with in their polemics. She had accepted their griping and sniping as both necessary and healthy, as much of an outlet for the frustration all of them felt with what they saw around them as Jay Grossman's and Steve Newman's pronounced interest in women was for each of them an affirmation of life and youth in the face of death and old age.

But lately the racial bickering on 3H had intensified and the sullenness of Mary Obakwanga, Sonya Craig, her unit clerk, Maria Ortez, and the aides on the day staff who made up the militant clique could no longer be overlooked. And though for a while nothing specific had happened to warrant comment or action, the head nurse had become convinced that for reasons of her own, Mary Obakwanga wanted to provoke a racial confrontation between them. Because of the quarrelsomeness of Walter Forsyth, it had come today.

On an absolute scale of values, however noisy and disgraceful, the scene between Mary Obakwanga and Walter Forsyth meant very little. Forsyth had not been endangered by the nurse's actions, only discomfited, and there was no question in Margaret Striker's mind that the African nurse had been well provoked. Evidently, Walter Forsyth could exasperate a saint, and Margaret Striker had no illusions anyone on her staff fit the ideal image of the nurse entertained by Sue Barton readers. She knew it was as easy to dislike Fosyth's brand of arrogance in someone who was sick as in someone who was well, but there were rules about expressing that dislike, and more rules governing a nurse's behavior. No excuse existed for Mary Obakwanga's deliberate disregard of Forsyth's call bell or for the ugly scene that had ensued, nor could the head nurse overlook insubordination to her own orders no matter how well she understood that the perfect compassion and the dispassionate composure required to handle a man like Forsyth were not easily combined. She was going to have to discipline Mary Obakwanga if only to assert her own authority, but it was not simple to decide what to do. To chastise her in private without making the reprimand "official," Margaret Striker knew, might be construed by the militants as an evidence of weakness on her part, but the head nurse also realized that if she chose to report the Rwandan nurse to her supervisors or place her officially on warning for unprofessional conduct, Mary Obakwanga's record would be smirched and she would be on probation so that any future incident might bring dismissal. Whatever move she made, she knew that there would be a reaction within the nursing staff and it was the form this reaction might take that concerned her now as much as the effect her decision would have on Mary Obakwanga.

"I don't know exactly how to handle this one," Margaret Striker confessed to Marie Velasquez when she found the assistant head nurse in the medications room a little while after leaving Tanya Olsen. "I'm going to have to talk about what happened with Obakwanga over with the supervisors you know—they're bound to hear about it upstairs anyway. But before I put in a call to Nancy Maxwell I'd like to know what you think, Marie. What reading do you get? As Mary goes so goes the gang?"

"I just don't know, Margaret," Marie Velasquez replied with a characteristic shrug of her shoulders, her hands lifted palms upward in a gesture of puzzlement. "I put myself on your side today when I tore into Obakwanga for neglecting Forsyth in the first place so the feedback has been pretty slow in coming this time. Have you picked up any vibes yourself?" she asked. "And what are you considering? Going to report her officially?"

"I can't decide what to do, Marie," the head nurse answered, pouring out a dose of Tylenol for herself to treat an incipient headache that inevitably followed the hives of tension already apparent at her throat.

"Because as dumb as this whole thing is—there's something in it that's queer—something I can't put my finger on that makes me believe that consciously or unconsciously, Obakwanga wanted this to happen. I think she needs to have a showdown with me so she can quit without losing face and if I duck the issue with Forsyth, I'm convinced there'll be scenes with her anyway. But I don't want to report her because I don't want to lose her if I can help it. We sure would be in trouble around here with only eight RNs to cover all twenty-one shifts a week and God knows when we'd get a replacement for her or what they'd send us. But on the other side of it, I can't let her get away with insubordination to orders or there'll be hell to pay on discipline and we've got enough trouble with some of the day group already. So I'm going to talk to Nancy, find out what the situation is with recruitment, and stall. Let Obakwanga stew tonight," she added wearily, glancing at her watch as she saw Marion Ping, the cheerful Philippine nurse on evening duty, making her way down the hall, surprised to see that it was already three o'clock. "I'll come to report late, act like a great stone face, and leave early. I've got paper work I want to do anyway for Dela Hanze—and then I'll sit down with Nancy and try to figure out how we can reprimand Obakwanga without giving her an excuse to quit. Ah . . ." she added, pulling a set of keys out of her pocket to unlock the narcotics cabinet and take out the log book in which, from shift to shift, a record of the stock and dispensation of every pain killer and tranquilizer was recorded, "the games we do play. Why in Christ's name can't Mary just say, 'I'm fed up—I want out'? We all are. We all *do* want out sometimes. I mean, you'd have to be crazy to *want* to stay in a place like this for very long."

Margaret Striker met Nancy Maxwell at O'Casey's, the small, seedy pub with its long, black oak bar and worn leatherette booths near the hospital frequented after hours by the house staff and nurses, at half past four. By half past five she had made a decision about Mary Obakwanga that surprised her.

A slight blonde whose round granny glasses emphasized a look of perpetual tiredness and seemingly permanent incredulity that was an appropriate reflection of the way the supervising nurse generally felt about her work, Nancy Maxwell had an uncanny way of helping the head nurses of the wards of which she was in charge to sort out their problems simply by listening to them and, though she rarely offered any direct advice, the supervisor's counsel was much prized by Margaret Striker and the others. Though Nancy Maxwell went about the hospital looking dazed, clutching her clipboards and notebooks to her chest, arms crossed, and losing her glasses, her cardigans and cigarette lighters with profligate regularity, despite her almost legendary absentmindedness, the supervisor seldom missed anything of human importance on her rounds and never failed to bring a kindly, crazy wisdom to bear on her nurses' difficulties that somehow always made sense and placed things in a calm perspective.

This afternoon, when she first slid into the booth opposite Margaret Striker, hunching up her omnipresent cardigan to keep it from slipping off her shoulders and pushing her blond hair back out of her eyes ineffectually, she began their conversation by ordering Margaret Striker to give her only good news.

"What good news?" the head nurse asked, smiling. "Did I ever ask you to meet me to bring you good news?"

"Tell me you're in love. I'm told by the grapevine you're in love. That would be good news."

"I'm in love," Margaret Striker said in jest to amuse her friend, but realized even as she said it that she told the truth.

"Are you really?" Nancy Maxwell asked, grinning crazily. "Oh, that's fine. That's therapeutic. That'll get you through at least six more months on your unit. Now you can tell me the bad news."

"I've got troubles with Obakwanga," Margaret Striker began, watching Nancy Maxwell fumble in her uniform pockets for a lighter that should have been there but was not. "I may have to put her on report."

"So what else is new?" Nancy Maxwell asked, now scratching in the recesses of her immense pocketbook for a match she finally uncovered and used to light her cigarette with a tremulous hand. "Only my thirty-sixth cigarette today," she mused absently, shaking a burning match to extinguish it. "Mary's been looking for a scrap with you for a month."

"You noticed?"

"I noticed."

"Do you think she *wants* a racial blowup?"

"Do you?" the supervisor asked, puffing hungrily and happily on the cigarette, her face almost obscured by smoke but beyond the look of incredulity, something shining in her eyes, keen and clever.

The story of Mary Obakwanga's quarrel with Walter Forsyth and her subsequent insubordination emerged piecemeal, interlarded with comments from Margaret Striker that revealed the head nurse's own confusions and the day's emotional stress. But as she neared the end of her account she heard herself saying, "So I *have* to report her. I have no other choice if I'm to maintain my authority. She'll quit anyway, I think. No matter what I do or don't do now, she'll find a way to quit over a racial question soon because she doesn't want to be caught giving up. But Mary's through here. Worn out by it. She's been on the floor for a year and something, and for most of it she's been living with that quasi revolution going on in her own country. She's got family in London and I think she'll go there. So I'll report her, but if she resigns I want a promise from you, Nancy, that nothing goes on her record. Let her save face too. After all, that's what I'm doing, isn't it?" she asked. Looking up from her glass of beer, she saw Nancy Maxwell, a maverick grin on her face, nodding vigorously. "Yuh," Margaret Striker continued then, affirming the answer to her own question, "that's what I'm doing. But I'll tell you something else, Nancy."

"What's that?" the supervisor asked, stretching herself back against the leatherette booth, relaxed now.

"I never liked Mary Obakwanga. Not really. And all afternoon I've been trying to figure out if that makes me a racist after all."

"And does it?"

"No," said Margaret Striker, feeling somewhat ridiculous but relieved, "because she didn't like me one little bit either."

"Right on," said Nancy Maxwell, fisting her hand and gesturing with it. "And does that make her a black racist?"

"Haven't the foggiest," Margaret Striker replied. "Maybe just human."

There was no answer from Nancy Maxwell. The supervisor sat quietly, studying Margaret Striker for a moment. Then, gathering up her many things, she said, "I'm glad you're in love. It's good for anybody. So now go sing and be at peace and at one with all the other nice people in your group who sing for that reason. And then take a hot bath tonight and sleep well."

"And you, Nancy?" Margaret Striker asked, getting up with the supervisor and helping her to gather the inevitable stack of books and papers she seemed always to carry about with her before the two walked out of the bar together into the twilight streets of the city, through which the sunset had run a seam of salamander-red that had lacquered the tenements and set the streets aflame. "What will you be doing while I'm at choir practice?"

"Oh, classes," said the supervisor, who was completing a masters degree by night while continuing, full time, in her job. "Classes and classes and classes and one day—in spring—it'll all be over."

Chapter 21

Tuesdays were always bad. Reacting to the data in lab reports that came back in the afternoon after the weekend hiatus late on Monday, the doctors invariably wrote new orders and scheduled a spate of tests for the next day. Accordingly, on Tuesday mornings Margaret Striker was in the habit of coming to 3H a little early to take a look at her books before hearing report and she usually arrived on the unit at a little before seven. But on this particular Tuesday such a snarl of orders had been written the previous evening that even prior to learning from the night nurse that Mary Obakwanga had called in sick, Margaret Striker knew that she would have to function more like a traffic controller than a nurse that day. Two patients scheduled for surgery were prepped and ready to go to the OR but a number of others were also to be sent off the floor during the morning. Mary O'Malley, the girl with the newly diagnosed Hodgkin's disease, was scheduled for lymphangiography. Dorita Volmer's cardiac catheterization had been moved from Thursday to nine that morning. Other patients were to be prepared for bronchoscopies, liver scans, a GI series, and a brain scan. The blood books were also heavily flagged with orders; twenty-six of the forty-two patients on the floor were to have blood samples drawn for lab work. While the interns were busy with this, the head nurse and the unit clerk would have to sort, label, and organize the specimens if they were to be ready in time for the morning lab pickup. Some orders, like those Mark Eaglesbury had written for Tanya Olsen, were particularly heavy. He had not only called for a complete blood count, hematocrit, and smear, repeating the workup that had been lost the previous evening, but had also ordered a full list of baseline tests on her blood including alkaline phosphates, serum creatinine, blood gases, electrolytes, complement levels, "sed" rates, BUN, and enzymes. Mrs. Olsen was also scheduled for a flat plate chest X-ray and an electrocardiograph that morning. Four of the heart patients on the floor were on monitors, eight diabetics would require blood sugar tests at intervals throughout the day, and Mr. Forsyth, on whom Dr. Richards had ordered a full list of baseline blood work, was down for a glucose tolerance test. The nurses were also keeping intake and output records on a dozen patients on fluid therapy and those with Foleys and NG tubes. Two of the leukemics on the floor were to receive whole pack transfusions that morning and the order books noted that Harold Blumenthal's Cryo would be sent up to be defrosted at nine.

The long list of orders confirmed that medicine as it was practiced on 3H relied heavily on tests and hardware, but it also hinted at something else Margaret Striker knew to be true, namely that in dealing with their patients what many of the medical staff preferred to see were not the fearful human beings who worried and wondered what was going on, but the factual test results which allowed them to reduce each patient to a medical problem and a manageable list of abstract questions and answers like those that had been implicit in the lab work done on Tanya Olsen the previous Thursday.

She had been seen that day in the clinic by Mark Eaglesbury and a hematologist who, suspecting leukemia, had sent a smear and a CBC to the blood lab. The results had revealed that Mrs. Olsen's white count was dangerously elevated at fifty-eight thousand, far in excess of the normal range of five to ten thousand. This finding and her other symptoms had dictated a specific response from the doctors, for it had told them that Mrs. Olsen was probably suffering from an acute form of leukemia and that she might be close to a crisis. They had therefore informed the stunned woman of her situation and recommended immediate hospitalization. Warning that intensive combination chemotherapy, the only available treatment for her disease, was experimental and required her consent, they indicated that though there were dangers attached to it, combination chemotherapy represented logical orderly attacks on her disease which were being studied for their comparative effectiveness against its various forms. Without neglecting to tell her that no cure for leukemia was yet known, both doctors stressed that remissions from her form of the disease were possible and left to Mrs. Olsen the decision whether to enter the hospital as an individual patient whose treatment program would be chosen by house staff, or as a member of a study group who would be cared for under a regimen dictated to her doctors according to protocols governing the leukemia research program. But they did not discuss with her in any detail the specific risks she might encounter during treatment nor did either doctor labor at length the fact that whatever happened to her, whether she lived or died, whether she suffered terribly during the period in which she submitted to an intentional poisoning of her bone marrow aimed at eradicating cancer cells from it, or whether she was fortunate enough not to experience any of the secondary effects of the disease and its treatment—bone pain, rampant infection, central nervous system destruction, thrombocytopenia, and hemorrhage—the results of her case would be meticulously reviewed for what they might reveal about the effectiveness of the combination of drugs used in treating her, even though the unmanageable question of what it meant to be Tanya Olsen in such a situation would scarcely be considered.

When the head nurse had looked into her room on her way in that morning at six forty-five, Mrs. Olsen had been lying absolutely still in her bed, her arms folded on her chest, her eyes fixed on the ceiling as they had been yesterday, and the head nurse had wondered just how much of what she had been told about her state Mrs. Olsen had actually understood. "How was Olsen last night?" she asked Helen Fisk, the night nurse, as she turned from the order books and Mark Eaglesbury's lengthy notes. "Did she seem particularly depressed to you?"

"Depressed!" Helen Fisk responded with emphasis. "Why, I think she's practicing to be dead! I went in three or four times last night," she said, falling in step beside the head nurse as the two walked toward the dialysis room at the end of the ward the nurses used for report, "and even though we had given her seconal I swear she didn't sleep a wink. Didn't move, either. Just lay there, staring at the ceiling like somebody with their eyes open in a coffin. I didn't stay with her long though because Mr. Forsyth was raisin' hell along with Mrs. Hanze."

"Dela was at it again last night, huh?" the head nurse asked without surprise as she pushed open the door to the dialysis to find several of the day nurses already assembled there. "But what about Forsyth? Was he hallucinating too?"

"No—I don't think that was it—though he sure was shouting and carrying on like a crazy man for a while," she answered, slumping into a chair next to Marie Velasquez. "No, he wasn't hallucinating. I'm sure of that. He knew just what was going on and then at about three o'clock he called me in there and tried to bribe me to make a bunch of long distance phone calls for him. Offered me a hundred dollars."

"And you took it?" Marie Velasquez looked up from her clipboard notes, laughing.

"No, man," Fisk answered her, grinning at her impishly, "but only 'cause I was too busy to make phone calls, you know that."

"Was he hallucinating then, do you think?" Margaret Striker asked soberly, "or did he mean it?"

"I think he meant it," Helen Fisk answered her. "He sure was urgent about it anyway. Wanted me to call Las Vegas, Miami, and—would you believe it—a place called Cartagena. Didn't he just come back from some place like that in South America? Isn't that where he got sick?"

"With reticulum cell sarcoma as his original underlying disease," Margaret Striker answered the LPN flatly, "he may have been sick before he ever went wherever it was he went last month. But evidently Mr. Forsyth is one of those cases of superdenial. He just won't believe he's going to die. He evidently thinks he's got malaria and has just dropped the possibility of metastatic sarcoma out of his mind completely, even though I'm told he was treated for it last spring, told his prognosis, and sent home on prednisone."

"What are they looking for now, Margaret?" Marie Velasquez asked. "Wasn't he controlled last spring?"

"I just don't know, Marie," the head nurse answered. "But I'll find out today. I've got him. Obakwanga called in sick."

There was a peculiar silence for a moment as the day nurse and aides absorbed this piece of information before Helen Fisk began giving her report at the head nurse's request. "In room 312," she began matter-of-factly, "Mr. Dix—scleraderma—is resting comfortably. Mr. Black is on penicillin Q four hours three million units IV; his temperature was 102 at four this morning. Mr. Brown is spilling 3+. Mr. O'Rourke complains of chest pain. He is on a monitor. He was clustering PVCs at one. In room 314 Miss O'Malley spent a quiet night. Mrs. Frazer, the same. In 316— Mrs. Suarez was on the monitor, resting comfortably, no complaints. Mrs. Olsen, no complaints."

After changeover rounds Margaret Striker went directly to 322 to give Dorita Volmer, one of the patients on her patient care list, medications before she was sent down for cardiac catheterization and found Dr. Richards, his face visibly bruised as a result of yesterday's altercation in the elevator, already with her, explaining the mechanics of the procedure in his most professional style.

"It'll be quite simple," he said reassuringly, standing before Mrs. Volmer, who sat in her wheelchair with needlework in her lap, staring up at him intently. "They'll just thread the catheter tip into the left ventrical arterially, visualizing it fluoroscopically as they move it up into the atrium. As it goes the catheter records pressures and samples the saturation of the blood, while flow patterns are recorded fluoroscopically by the use of an indicator substance, usually a radio opaque contrast medium. They'll be watching particularly for mitral regurgitants and, as you've been told, for the effects of aortic stenosis and possible left ventricular hypertrophy."

This was, the head nurse knew, an adequate description of the mechanics of the procedure the surgeons would employ to probe the anomalies of Mrs. Volmer's heart that morning, and to the extent that Dr. Richards at least admitted the woman's right to know what was going to happen to her, the intern's performance

130

was preferable to some the head nurse had seen given in comparable situations by physicians who chose to treat their patients as witless children. But it was a *performance* nevertheless—one meant as much to impress Mrs. Volmer with the mysterious cleverness of her doctors as it was to reassure her, and it was obvious to the head nurse as she studied the woman's reactions to Richards' deliberately difficult language that though Mrs. Volmer was trying hard to follow the meaning of what she was being told, she had only the haziest notion of what the intern's words really meant but was embarrassed to ask for a simpler explanation because she did not want to appear ignorant and was afraid to seem to doubt the young doctor.

A scene like this belonged to a genre that had always disturbed the head nurse not only because it left someone like Mrs. Volmer unnecessarily bewildered but because it had the effect of placing even an inexperienced physician like Frank Richards in the role of a shaman whose rites were beyond common understanding. Though it was often argued that promoting the patients' faith in the doctors saved them useless anxiety and helped to sustain their courage, Margaret Striker had too often seen this rationale used to rob patients and their families of their rights to be consulted on matters of profound importance to them. It was simpler, much of the time, for a physician to make a unilateral medical decision on a case than to take the time to explain his intentions to his patients, and on a floor as busy as 3H the interns and residents were sometimes driven to do so by the sheer pressure of events.

But keeping patients ignorant of the risks they faced not only fostered the blind belief that physicians could work miracles, but, supported by precisely the kind of reluctance to ask questions Mrs. Volmer was presently exhibiting, certain doctors were encouraged to assume an absolute authority in their dealings with patients that was unjustified on 3H where the practice of medicine was as flawed as its all-too-human practitioners.

When Dr. Richards concluded his performance by patting Mrs. Volmer paternally on the shoulder and assuring her that the surgeons would go through it all again downstairs, he asked Mrs. Volmer with apparent sincerity if she had any questions. Predictably, though for a moment she seemed to hesitate nervously on the verge of asking him something, she did not, and after glancing at his watch the intern was swiftly gone.

"Did you understand all that?" Margaret Striker, who had been making up her bed, asked Mrs. Volmer quietly as soon as the intern had left the room, "or can I help you with any of it?"

Mrs. Volmer fumbled with her needlework for a moment, a pattern of tiger lilies cross stitched on a pillowcase, before she replied, "Well, they're going to stick a needle into my heart, aren't they, to find out what's the matter with it?"

It took the head nurse ten minutes more to explain to Dorita Volmer how the catheter—a flexible, wire-thin tubing—would be threaded with infinite care through the blood vessels back into her heart's left chambers to take samples of the blood and explore its pressures and flow patterns to help measure the degree of stenosis, or thickening of the valve openings of her heart due to the calcification of scar tissue evidently left on them in the wake of a childhood bout of rheumatic fever. When she emerged from Mrs. Volmer's room and headed toward Harold Blumenthal's, Margaret Striker had a distinct sense of accomplishment in knowing that at least at this point in the events that seemed to be propelling the attractive fifty-two-year-old grandmother toward heart surgery, Mrs. Volmer understood exactly what was going on, and that though she was not without apprehension neither was she mystified. "So today will decide it," she had said to the head nurse as she prepared to leave 322. "Today they'll know what is wrong with my heart. Will they tell me, do you think?"

"Only if you ask them," Margaret Striker had answered her, "and only if you really want to know. . . ."

"Oh—I think I want to know," Mrs. Volmer had said stoically. "Or rather that I *have* to know, even though I suspect it won't make much difference in my decision. You see, as things are now I can't even fly kites on the beach with my grandchildren."

Chapter 22

Kate Blaine and Margaret Striker had just finished hanging the first transfusion pack of antihemophilic globulin for Mr. Blumenthal when a group of hematologists, led by Dr. Dorothy Blackmur, one of the luminaries of the hospital's medical staff, crowded into room 324, trailed by Steve Newman and Mark Eaglesbury.

Dr. Blackmur, a steely-haired woman in her early fifties, enjoyed an impressive reputation among the house staff as a teacher and diagnostician, but to her patients, most of whom were leukemics, she was more like a god. Frank James, the cellist who had recently undergone a second course of intensive chemotherapy on 3H and won a remission, had claimed that Dr. Blackmur had an artist's ability to perceive at a glance the precise physical and emotional state of her patients. But while it seemed more likely to the head nurse that the meticulous follow-ups Dr. Blackmur insisted on with her patients had as much to do with her diagnostic genius as unfettered intuition, from where Margaret Striker had stood at the bedside of several dozens of leukemics over the past three years, Dorothy Blackmur's reputation was well earned. With literally hundreds of leukemics in her care, Blackmur followed through with each one doggedly, win or lose, from the beginning of treatment to its end, and her arrival on 3H that morning heartened the head nurse. For if Blackmur intended to make rounds on Tanya Olsen, as Mark Eaglesbury's presence in her entourage indicated, it seemed probable that she would take charge of her case. And though Margaret Striker entertained little hope for Mrs. Olsen, the nurse knew that as one of Blackmur's patients she would receive every chance there was.

Coming into 324, Dr. Blackmur greeted Walter Forsyth but did not stop at his bedside. Instead, she went directly to Harold Blumenthal's, motioning the group to follow. "How are you feeling, Harold?" she asked him familiarly, as her minions grouped around her in a semicircle, every one of the research fellows, all of them men, quite unconsciously imitating the woman's slouch-shouldered stance. "Not too good from the look of things. Still bleeding? Well—don't get in too much of a fuss," she continued easily, "Dr. Newman and Dr. Blaine know what they're doing and I'll be keeping in touch myself, as well as your very special friend, Dr. Gaffney. The four of us should be able to manage to get you a percentage gain and send you home soon. Okay?"

"How soon and for how long?" Blumenthal asked her, his brown eyes keen despite the grayish pallor of his face. "I need ninety days to make up my Medicare. Will you sign on the dotted line for ninety days at home?"

"Ninety it'll be," she assured him, turning then to Kate Blaine and motioning toward the door. "I know you're reporting to Gaffney first, Dr. Blaine," she said in a voice of quiet but unmistakable authority. "Mr. Blumenthal is not officially my patient, but we've been keeping tabs on him in our unit as well and I want the facts. See that we get the percentage gains, if any, this afternoon, to-night, tomorrow—and for as long as you continue this course of treatment. If you go to cytotoxics I want to know," she continued, turning to Newman as she moved briskly down the hall at the head of the wedge of doctors. "The same on Forsyth. Keep us informed. He was on the protocol last spring and we'll follow through. Now—who's next? Olsen, isn't it?" she asked in a busi-nesslike voice, fishing an index card out of her white coat pocket. "A new admission tentatively AML?"

Falling in line behind the phalanx, Margaret Striker, though not finished in 324, nevertheless followed the doctors across the ward to 316 and stood unobtrusively at the back of the group as Blackmur halted them just outside Mrs. Olsen's door.

"What's the count?" she demanded of Mark Eaglesbury. "And I'll want to look at yesterday's smear myself."

"I'm sorry, Doctor," Eaglesbury murmured, embarrassed, "but the stat bloods were lost last night. I sent another set this morn-ing."

"Stat?" she asked.

134

"No, I'm sorry," he stammered.

"Never mind," she said. "You were on last night, I take it. Well, they won't be ready yet, then. Tell me what you *do* know."

"Well," Mark Eaglesbury began nervously, "Mrs. Olsen was seen first in clinic last Thursday on a direct referral from her private physician. He had seen her twice in the last six weeks. She was complaining of fatigue, random pains in her arms, legs, and elsewhere, and an increasing sense of malaise. Blood counts taken twice showed elevated WBCs, high enough the last time to call for the referral. On Thursday the white count was fifty-eight thousand and I ordered a smear. We found blasts and the stain also showed myelocytes and promyelocytes. Her platelet count was depressed—seventy-two hundred—and hemoglobin was fourteen. We admitted her as an elective for this morning. I've started a D5W IV and ordered platelets, pending final diagnosis. I sent a six and twelve channel this morning and a repeat stat CBC, smear, and need a marrow aspiration."

"Thank you, Doctor," Blackmur responded tonelessly as she led the group into 316, where Tanya Olsen, who was dozing, lay with the sheets drawn up and perfectly folded across her breast, her complexion, in sleep, paste-colored.

"Mrs. Olsen," Dr. Blackmur said softly, drawing the lavender curtain around the cubicle and pulling a chair up next to the bed as Tanya Olsen stirred into wakefulness to find herself surrounded by people in white. "Mrs. Olsen, I am Dr. Blackmur, one of the senior hematologists in this hospital, and I am the specialist in charge of your case. . . . Now, I would like to know all I can about you," she continued, reaching up her hand into which one of her research fellows put a clipboard already countaining the pertinent lab slips from the clinic and a copy of the intern's and resident's admission notes on Mrs. Olsen. "I want to know how you have felt in the past few months, when you first began to feel fatigued, what you have been told by the doctors, and what you understand of what you have been told. But I also want to know about you personally, your family background, your parents, children. . . ."

It was an artful interview and by the time it was over Dorothy Blackmur had not only extracted an orderly history from Tanya Olsen, but she had explained to her the lethal mechanics of her disease in clear, concise, and strangely unemotional and untechnical language that stood in marked contrast to the abstruse terms Frank Richards had employed this morning to describe cardiac catheterization to Dorita Volmer.

"I don't know how much the doctors have told you already about leukemia," she had begun simply, "but at the risk of repeating them, I'm going to tell you about it because I feel it is essential that you understand.

"Your body," she continued matter-of-factly when Mrs. Olsen made no response except to turn her head so that she could look at Dr. Blackmur directly as the hematologist spoke, "is constantly producing and using up blood, which is manufactured in the marrow of the bones. Healthy marrow produces red cells, which are responsible for transporting oxygen, and white cells, which are responsible for protecting the body against infection, and platelets. Platelets are very specialized blood cells that keep you from bleeding. All three are produced by normal marrow in amounts that meet your body's needs—almost as if the marrow were programmed to do so. Well, in leukemia the 'programming'—if you will allow us to use that term—becomes confused and unhealthy marrow manufactures only one kind of cell—a white blood cell that is in itself abnormal in the sense that it is immature and unable to do its primary job of fighting infection. These immature white cells—we call them 'blasts'—soon become so packed into the marrow that they crowd out whatever healthy marrow is left and begin to spill out into the bloodstream, where, as in the marrow, they crowd out healthy blood cells and eventually invade the various organs of the body. The result is anemia, producing the kind of fatigue you have been experiencing, possible internal bleeding or bleeding at the skin's surface, which produces the kind of bruising you have shown in the past week, some pain—not unlike arthritic pain—and a low threshold for infection. These are the secondary effects of leukemia and these are things we can treat.

"But we can also treat the primary problem," Dr. Blackmur went on, undeterred by Mrs. Olsen's withdrawn silence. "We have ways of destroying the abnormal blast cells, of eradicating them in the marrow and elsewhere in the body so that healthy marrow has a chance to come back and replace unhealthy marrow. . . . Now," she said firmly, standing up and beginning to pace back and forth in the narrow space at Mrs. Olsen's bedside, holding her hand up to her face in a characteristic gesture of thoughtfulness that gave emphasis to her words, "there *is* risk in this treatment, risk that thus far we have not been able to eliminate. Sometimes we cannot overcome the leukemia with our armaments and sometimes we cannot supply sufficient protection against infection and bleeding. I should also add," she continued, "that certain kinds of leukemia are more difficult to attack than others. But your form, if the diagnosis of acute myelocytic leukemia holds up in today's lab work, is one of the forms with which we have had some success in up to one third of the samples we have studied."

"There is a chance for me?" Mrs. Olsen asked then, in a flat voice that sounded almost sleepy. "A one-third chance to live?" she asked, turning her head again to fix her pale eyes on Dr. Blackmur's and lifting her right hand in a weary gesture of acquiescence.

"I cannot be that precise," Dr. Blackmur answered her honestly, pausing in her pacing. "I would have to check the statistics in terms of your age, sex, and any number of factors to be precise. . . ."

"A one-third chance to live, maybe, then," said Tanya Olsen quietly, looking back at the ceiling. "And a two-thirds chance to die . . . I didn't expect it, you see," she added, dropping her hand down at her side again. "Not at all."

"None of us do—ever," Dr. Blackmur answered in almost a murmur. "At least not at first." Then, seating herself again, the hematologist resumed her unemotional tone. "Now. Once we de-

137

termine your precise diagnosis you will be put on a protocol. The course of treatment to which you will be assigned, though it will be appropriate to your form of leukemia, will be chosen at random from several possible courses and combinations of drugs. As I believe has been explained to you, Mrs. Olsen, we do not yet know which combination of drugs *is* the most effective and the protocols are designed to help us find out by making comparisons on a nationwide scale that will eventually give us that information. But whatever protocol you are put on, be assured that every drug on it, by itself, has proven effective to a degree. Our problem is not finding the right drugs per se—though we continue to search for newer, better forms—but in finding the best *combination* of drugs."

"And my problem," Tanya Olsen said almost inaudibly, turning her gaze back to Dr. Blackmur, tears in her eyes, "is whether I die now or later, isn't it?"

Dr. Blackmur, her own expression suddenly clouding, closed her eyes and nodded. "Yes, Mrs. Olsen. That is true." She rose from her chair almost wearily. "But if you wish to take the chance we offer, I promise you I will do my very best for you." Then, reaching down, she took Tanya Olsen's hand firmly in her own and said, "You may of course rescind the consent for treatment under the protocols you have given us and choose not to become part of the overall study. We will treat you in any case—if you so wish—beginning today. But know this much—whether you join the study group under the protocols or not, we will try to help you. If you are in the study, though Eaglesbury and Newman will be your doctors, they will both be reporting directly to me and I myself will see you regularly. If you do not, you will be their patient, but they will still be governed by our advice and work, so that whichever choice you make, I will still be seeing you from time to time. If at any time you feel you must see me you need only to ask and I will try to visit you as soon as I can. I promise you that." She studied Mrs. Olsen's face for a moment, searching it with a gentleness in her own face that was more eloquent than words, and then, trailed by her silent entourage, she left, leaving only the head nurse standing at the foot of the bed, behind the pale purple curtain, watching Tanya Olsen as she began to cry silently.

"She meant it," the nurse said, trying to give reassurance. "She will try to help you and she's a very, very fine doctor. And I promise you, we too will try. We will always be here when you need us."

"Only God can help me now," Tanya Olsen answered her gently, looking straight into Margaret Striker's eyes. "And though I see His goodness shining in your face, there is nothing anyone can *do* for me. I know that and so do you." She was silent but the nurse, feeling something like pain tightening in her throat, remained for a moment where she was, unable to move or speak. Then, after a long sigh, Tanya Olsen asked. "How old are you?"

"I'm twenty-six," Margaret Striker answered.

"And I'm fifty-two. Just twice your age. I don't even know what happened to the years in between. . . ."

Chapter 23

Not until the lull that usually occurred between the hours of ten-twenty and eleven-thirty, after she had made rounds of the ward with Marie Velasquez to check vital signs, was Margaret Striker able to return to 324 to resume her patient assignment. She had expected to find Mr. Forsyth in a rage by that time, but in her absence Dr. Richards had started his glucose tolerance test and, placated by this attention, Forsyth, absorbed by the activity in Mr. Blumenthal's cubicle, diagonally opposite his, was subdued and almost amiable.

"Harold's a very sick man, isn't he?" Forsyth asked the nurse as she began remaking his bed for him, rolling his bulk from side to side carefully so that the IV line implanted in his left arm did not pull loose.

"What has he told you?" the head nurse asked him guardedly, unwilling to betray confidential information about one patient to another.

"He's been explaining to me that he's a hemophiliac," Forsyth replied, "and that he's in big trouble because he's resistant to the stuff they can give him to stop his bleeding inside."

"That's true," Margaret Striker responded, "but they expect to help him."

"They helped me," Forsyth said then. "Last year I was dying and they cured me."

"Oh? Of what?" the head nurse asked, probing delicately to see just how much about his underlying sarcoma Forsyth accepted and how much he denied.

"Cancer. I had cancer last year and they cured me. X-rays, chemotherapy. I had it all and I got better."

"You went into remission?" the nurse asked carefully. "Is that what they told you?"

"No," Forsyth said roughly, "I'm cured. They stopped it. Wiped it out."

"Weren't you put on some kind of maintenance afterward though, Mr. Forsyth—to protect you? Didn't you continue taking certain drugs?"

"Yes, prednisone and something else—alla something."

"Allopurinol?"

"Yes, prednisone and allopurinol. That was to keep the cancer from coming back, you see. But I'm cured. No doubt about it. What's the matter with me now is that I picked up malaria down in South America, but these goddamned kid doctors here won't admit it."

"Oh?" the nurse replied noncommittally, wondering how Forsyth had arrived at so specific an explanation for the fatigue and intermittent fever listed in her card index file as FUO—a fever of unknown origin—which were his chief complaints and which were suspected of having a connection with his underlying sarcoma and the steroid therapy he had been receiving for the past five months to depress the spread of his disease that might also have encouraged an evolving diabetes. "How did you learn you had malaria?"

"A doctor in Cartagena told me," Forsyth answered readily. "He got it right away. Not like these idiot kids here, sticking me with needles. He put me on aspirin. . . ."

"He did?" the nurse asked, alarmed by the medical implications of this piece of information which indicated that Forsyth might also have experienced a number of slow internal bleeds as the dangerous combination of aspirin with the steroid, prednisone, had slowly worn away the clotting capacity of his blood. "Weren't you taking prednisone? Hadn't the doctors warned you never to take aspirin when you were on steroids?"

"Sure," said Forsyth, heaving himself up to a sitting position with the head nurse's help, "but I'd stopped taking that stuff after I got malaria. I was off it entirely in the Bahamas anyway."

"Bahamas?" the nurse asked, confused by Mr. Forsyth's peregrinations but also distracted by this second revelation, which might indicate that Forsyth's "malaria" had in fact been a reaction to a sudden withdrawal from prednisone. "I'm confused, Mr. Forysth. I thought you saw the doctor in Cartagena and that he told you to take aspirin for your fever. Did he also tell you then to stop taking the prednisone?" she queried, realizing that this sequence of events had medical importance and might have slipped by the doctors. "I mean, were you taking them simultaneously or did you stop the prednisone before you took the aspirin or what? I don't really understand how we got from Cartagena to the Bahamas just now—or rather, I don't know why."

"Look, stupid," Forsyth replied without rancor, "I'm a gambler. That's what I do for a living now; I gamble. I was in Vegas. I went from there to Cartagena—like I told you. I vomited. I got a fever. I started taking aspirin. I went to the doctor and he said I probably had malaria but that the aspirin was good for fever. I finished up my business, but I still felt pretty lousy so I thought I oughta get out of Cartagena. It's hot as hell there anyway. I went to the Bahamas and that was when I lost some of my bags. That steroid stuff was in the bags they lost, so I didn't have it to take anymore. Anyway, I kept feeling worse in the Bahamas so I finally came up here."

"Mr. Forsyth, why didn't you come straight back to New York when you first began to feel ill? Hadn't the doctors told you to keep in close touch with them? Hadn't they explained that it was very important for you to stay on your medications?"

"And didn't I tell you gambling is how I make my living?" Forsyth responded, suddenly on guard and hostile. "I had business down there. Business that's nobody's business. People I had to see. I came back when I could."

At the nursing station Margaret Striker took Walter Forsyth's chart out of the rack and read swiftly through the admitting notes written the previous evening by the assistant resident, Jay Grossman, and intern Richards. Though neither made any direct mention of what Forsyth had just told her about combining aspirin with steroids, there was evidence in both doctors' assessments of Forsyth's present condition that they knew he had gone off the maintenance regimen dictated for sarcoma patients by the protocols and each noted that a steroid-withdrawal reaction could have contributed to his recent malaise. But beyond this the head nurse found herself absorbed by other things Forsyth's chart revealed about him and his reaction to his illness.

Forsyth had come to the hospital in April, complaining of extreme fatigue and pain in his lower abdomen. A biopsy of swollen lymph nodes had yielded the diagnosis of reticulum cell sarcoma and lymphangiography, which allowed inspection by X-ray camera of the entire lymph system, had located matted masses of these cancerous cells in the groin, and around the sheath of the aorta—the great artery that rises from the heart and carries blood to the body. Treated by a combination of localized radiotherapy and generalized chemotherapy, the latter following a protocol being tested for sarcoma and intended to reach any undetected cancerous sites and eradicate them as radiotherapy had been used to destroy specific primary sites, Forsyth had been released from the hospital in May "in remission" and placed on a maintenance program of chemotherapy, one of the forty per cent of patients with this kind of cancer for whom the treatment had been relatively effective, who with careful management might expect to live, symptom-free, for another two to five years.

After his discharge Forsyth was seen regularly for the first six weeks by doctors at the clinic as part of his follow-up care, but by July he had become capricious about keeping his appointments and, according to the chart notes, had evidently resumed his free-style life, stepping up its pace, jetting from Las Vegas to Miami and from there to the fleshpots of the Caribbean with erratic frequency. He had seen his doctors only intermittently during this period. Claiming that he no longer needed them, he had boasted of living "high," of gambling for big stakes and winning, of eating and drinking and whoring heavily, a man in such a rage to live that in trying to outrun the shadow of death he had chosen deliberately to ignore the rules, regulations, appointments, medications, and warnings of the doctors who would force him to recognize the specter that followed him so closely and had instead begun killing himself slowly and willfully by excess. In time Forsyth's mistreatment of his body, weakened by his underlying disease and the powerful steroids he still took to keep it in check, began to tell. His liver became enlarged, whether as a result of alcohol or cancer no one yet knew. It also seemed likely now that a latent diabetes had become full blown in the last month. If uncontrolled it could have been responsible for the weakness, sweats, nervousness, and nausea Forsyth had reported experiencing sporadically before the onset of his fever equally as much as could infection, cirrhosis of the liver, irregular usage of steroids, a slow intermittent hemorrhage, chronic renal insufficiency, or any combination of these, and other possibilities. And to further perplex the doctors, the specific origin of Forsyth's reported fever was not known and they could not find any localized abscess or infection to explain it. But beneath all these particular questions Richards, Grossman, and Newman presently had to consider in asking themselves about Forsyth was the final one of whether he had suffered a relapse and whether the sarcoma that had been controlled in the spring had begun to spread itself, invading his liver, his lungs, his kidneys, and even the vertebrae of his backbone.

With a shudder Margaret Striker put his chart back on the rack and turned to the order books, disturbed by what she had read and by the ugly premonition that Walter Forsyth, arrogant, massive, outrageous, the passionate gambler who had fought for life by hurling himself into it, had wasted his strength trying to bluff death and now lay dying, piecemeal.

Chapter 24

Test results from the blood and electrolyte workups, from microbacteriology for culture reports, from serology and even from the special procedures done in the morning usually started to filter back to the ward just after lunch, and one of the first to be received, only moments before she herself was brought back to the floor on a stretcher, contained what seemed to be good news for Dorita Volmer. Though the surgeons had found considerable scar tissue narrowing the aortic valve which controls the flow of blood being pushed from the heart's left side to the body and brain, the results of the catheterization paired with an earlier angiogram did not seem to warrant replacing the damaged valve. Mrs. Volmer, evidently taking the place of a patient with a ventricular aneurysm who had died before his scheduled Thursday operation, was to undergo a closed-heart procedure in two days, during which the surgeons expected to ream open the narrow valve with a knife or even a finger, without actually opening the heart. A simpler operation, it entailed less risk than open heart surgery. But after this one piece of rather encouraging news, most of the rest of the results returned to 3H intermittently from one-thirty onward proved distressing.

Standing in for her unit clerk, who had gone to the dentist after lunch, Margaret Striker had taken a number of the earlier calls, giving lab results herself. Two of the first she had received had been Walter Forsyth's. His blood cultures, though as yet indeterminate, had turned up some microbes that might have caused his intermittent fevers, and his glucose tolerance test revealed significantly elevated blood-sugar levels for an extended period during the test, confirming that he was a diabetic. But the head nurse had no sooner notified Dr. Richards of these reports than both phones again began ringing simultaneously.

"Is Blaine around?" Marie Velasquez had asked after picking up one as Margaret Striker had answered the other. "It's about Blumenthal. Only a two point three per cent gain . . ."

"Oh, shit," said Margaret Striker flatly, already busily jotting down numbers on a scrap of paper that had upset her. "Take the full message. She'll be right back. . . . Yes, I got it, WBC seventy thousand," she repeated aloud after the lab technician on the other end of the line who had found the figures she was giving the head nurse sufficiently alarming to warrant calling them up to the ward immediately, "Platelets thirteen hundred—"

"My God," said Marie Velasquez, reacting to these numbers with as much dismay as the head nurse had to her terse report on Harold Blumenthal's poor reaction to the Cryo, "who's that?"

"It's Olsen," said Margaret Striker glumly, putting down the phone and pushing the intercom button to page Mark Eaglesbury. "Her white count is skyrocketing. She's either gotten wildly infected or is on the edge of blastic crisis. . . . Oh, Mark," she told the intern as he trotted up to the desk, mildly displeased to have been called from Newman's office, where he had been listening to Jay Grossman's latest tale of sexual conquest, "it's Mrs. Olsen. The white count is way up and the bottom seems to have dropped out of her platelets before you gave her those this morning. It's her CBC. I thought you'd want to know immediately."

Eaglesbury blanched visibly as he examined the scrap of paper the nurse shoved toward him on which she had scribbled Tanya Olsen's complete blood counts. Her white count now stood at 70,000, as compared to Thursday's reading of 58,000, and before

145

the morning's transfusion her platelet level had dropped to 1,300 —far below the normal limits of 150,000 to 450,000.

"Jesus, she's not spiking, is she?" the intern asked, clearly as worried as the head nurse by the evidence that Tanya Olsen was producing white cells at an accelerating rate that could indicate the onset of sepsis or even of a blastic crisis, as deformed leukocytes began literally to block up the smaller blood vessels, leaving major organs, the brain, and even her bones starving for oxygen. "She didn't spike a temperature this morning without my being told, did she? What about the cultures? Did we get them too? And the smear? Does Blackmur have it or what?"

"Look, Mark. There were no special orders on Mrs. Olsen's vital signs so we checked them at eight and ten. She wasn't spiking then. Her temperature was only slightly elevated—as it was on admission. I'll check her again now, but while I do that why don't you get on the horn and find out if they've pulled a protocol for her yet. If they haven't, tell 'em why you think they'd better hurry up. Do you want me to page Newman for you or do you want to hear the differentials first from the hematology lab?"

"No. I'll call Blackmur's section first, then talk to Newman. But will you check her for me right away? She could have spiked a fever. What's the hematology number?" he asked, pawing through the hospital telephone book ineffectually and impatiently.

"The lab technician's number is 7535," she answered, picking up an IVAC and moving briskly toward 316, pushing the manometer before her to check Tanya Olsen's blood pressure as well as her vital signs. "And Blackmur is 0065."

Tanya Olsen was apparently asleep, but at Margaret Striker's touch her eyes fluttered open and she stared up into the head nurse's eyes with the look of someone swimming upward from shadowed depths toward the light. She sighed deeply as the nurse fixed the blood pressure cuff in place.

"Does that hurt?" Margaret Striker asked solicitously, aware that Mrs. Olsen's oxygen-starved muscles and bones might be painfully sensitive.

"Some," Tanya Olsen replied in a whisper, closing her eyes again, apparently exhausted. "It aches. I ache."

The nurse did not answer, but as she listened with her stethoscope for the thud of Tanya Olsen's blood pushing out from her heart and the quiet that followed as the aortic valve closed in the diastolic phase of the heartbeat she was simultaneously studying Tanya Olsen's face. Even paler than she had been this morning, her eyelids now seemed almost a transparent white. But there was no significant fever, her pulses and respiration were steady and strong, and the blood pressures, though somewhat depressed, also were in normal ranges. Pulling the probe out of the IVAC, Margaret Striker inserted it gently between Mrs. Olsen's lips and held it in place for the fraction of a minute it took the highly sensitive machine to record a temperature. It was barely elevated at 100.1°, just above what is clinically normal. There was no clearcut sign yet of either approaching sepsis or of blastic crisis, but time was surely growing short.

Mark Eaglesbury was still on the phone when Margaret Striker got back to the nursing station with this report but the look he gave the head nurse signaled that the smear results he had just heard confirmed her own intuitive assessment of Tanya Olsen's precarious state. "She's got wildly deformed and immature cells all over the place—megaloblasts, myeloblasts, promyeloblasts. I'm on to Blackmur's office now. They've just about finished the randomization that will turn up her protocol and they're willing to give me the first part of it now and then send the complete copy up through the tubes."

Pulling a card from his white jacket pocket, the intern began jotting notes: "Number 7221," he repeated as he began taking down the first course of drugs he would administer under the protocol that had been selected at random for Tanya Olsen from among those designed to treat acute myelocytic leukemia. "Regimen D—Daunomycin, Cytosine, and Thioguanine . . ." A stunned, stricken look flickered in his usually impassive face momentarily as he intoned, "Given simultaneously . . ."

"Oh, Jesus," Margaret Striker later remembered saying, "it's the red death."

The protocols used to treat the various leukemias all were of differing strengths and combined poisons of many degrees of toxicity and speed of impact, but among those presently being tested, the protocol including Daunomycin had earned the title of "the red death" among the nurses because of the color of this drug and the potency of the combination. Employing some of the strongest cytotoxics in use—Cytosine and Thioguanine—the red death was immensely effective in eradicating cancerous cells in the bone marrow and bloodstream. But unfortunately these powerful drugs also destroyed healthy as well as cancerous blood cells, stripping the body of its defense against infection, and Daunomycin had a second undesirable quality of cardiotoxicity. Poisonous to the heart muscle, it could precipitate lethal arrhythmias.

"Well, she's in for it," Mark Eaglesbury said unemotionally, putting down the phone. "But, if she's got any chance at all for remission, this protocol will give it to her."

"If it doesn't kill her first," Margaret Striker answered unhappily. "This one throws everything at her at once. She'll have no resistance left whatsoever and I'm willing to bet right now that she's got something cooking to cause this tiny fever. . . ."

"Look, Margaret, I didn't design this protocol. If you don't like it, why don't you object to Blackmur?" Mark Eaglesbury answered snappishly. "I've been on for thirty hours straight now, so I'm not about to waste any of what's left of my energy on a useless discussion, so do you mind if we get started! Obviously I'll cover her against infection with an antibiotic, if it's necessary," he continued, gruff and businesslike, "but for now I want to get the poisons going. We gave her Compazine at noon, right? And there's a line in?"

"You asked us to put her on D5 and W to KVO this morning after the platelets, Doctor," the head nurse answered calmly. "And if you ordered Compazine, obviously we gave it. But I'll have to see if there's any Daunomycin on the floor," she added, heading toward the medications room. "Otherwise it'll take half an hour to get up here from the pharmacy."

Margaret had no wish to quarrel with the intern about Tanya Olsen's protocol; Mark Eaglesbury's testy response to her remark indicated that the intern, like herself, was dismayed that Mrs. Olsen had been assigned to one of the riskier combinations of drugs, even though he plainly resented being questioned about it by the nurse. For despite the fact that Mark Eaglesbury, like most young doctors, was zealous in his professed faith in medicine and would argue heatedly in defense of study programs like those being conducted by Blackmur and other researchers as necessary to producing knowledge which might one day provide an effective, low-risk approach to controlling leukemia and other cancers, he was not, as were too many other interns Margaret Striker had known, incapable of self-doubt or driven by such a need to succeed that he could not accept the idea of failure. Dr. Eaglesbury, in fact, had lately been heard to express a notion to which most nurses ascribed—that it was sometimes preferable to let a patient die with dignity than to prolong life at the price of destroying the individual. He had even gone so far as to argue with Jay Grossman publicly that doctors were hung up on death and sometimes subjected patients to cruel suffering, keeping them alive at any costs, for reasons that had more to do with saving their own egos than with saving the patients' lives. But in treating Tanya Olsen, Mark Eaglesbury was as much constrained by the prescribed course of treatment to which his patient had been assigned as Margaret Striker would be by his orders.

The protocol called for three drugs to be given simultaneously in the initial dosage—Daunomycin to be administered by injection directly into the vein, Cytosine to be given by intravenous infusion, and Thioguanine by mouth. For five days afterward Cytosine and Thioguanine would be repeated every twelve hours and the effects of the marrow production tracked by daily blood counts and when necessary by marrow aspirations. Within twenty-four hours, as the powerful poisons all but destroyed her body's

149

ability to produce its own blood supply, Tanya Olsen would become almost wholly dependent on the red blood cells, white cells, and platelets in circulation in her bloodstream. Shortest-lived of the three, the platelets would begin to disappear from circulation first, opening the way to generalized hemorrhaging, but in the next few days the hazards of hemorrhage would be no greater than those of infection. With the body's defenses against viral, bacterial, or fungal infestation already profoundly depressed by leukemia, as the white blood cells were all but wiped out by the poisons, her vulnerability to infection would increase dangerously.

While the doctors scanned the daily lab work for counts and cultures that would keep them informed of Tanya Olsen's progress—or the lack of it in the abstract—the nurses would be responsible for monitoring her physical condition hour by hour for any forewarning of the onset of infection. To support her meanwhile she would require transfusions both of platelets and of packed red blood cells as the condition of her blood indicated that these were necessary, with the greatest predictable need occurring when her marrow production could be expected to be at a standstill at the end of the poisons' course in five days. But, though both Margaret Striker and Mark Eaglesbury recognized the unfortunate timing involved, neither spoke of the fact that Tanya Olsen would be most endangered over the weekend. Instead, working with extreme caution—for the powerful drugs if given too quickly could produce life-threatening reactions, tissue burns and lesions—the head nurse and the intern began giving them at two o'clock, Eaglesbury injecting the Daunomycin into Tanya Olsen's vein as Margaret Striker, using the intravenous route already established, switched the line to the Cytosine mixed with normal saline solution and began timing its flow. As they worked they both chatted quietly with Tanya Olsen, who, buoyed by Compazine, spoke euphorically of going to see her daughter off on a cruise the following Sunday.

Chapter 25

On Wednesday morning, despite a dramatic drop in her white count from seventy thousand to three thousand, Tanya Olsen was holding her own against any latent infection. Her early vital signs continued on a straight line across the charts, all well within normal range, and the fractionally elevated temperature that had worried the head nurse on Tuesday had dropped to a steady 98.9 —all of which seemed to justify the cautiously optimistic attitude the head nurse assumed toward her that morning as she turned her energies to other, more immediate concerns. Since Mary Obakwanga had again called in sick Margaret Striker was once again carrying double duty—running the ward as head nurse and taking responsibility for six patients as well—and from report onward, because Marie Velasquez, who was to cover 3H over the weekend, had the day off, she was kept moving at such a clip that, though she would have liked to follow through with Tanya Olsen personally, it was impossible.

The problems list for the morning seemed inordinately long, and while it was perfectly plain from Helen Fisk's report that Dr. Blaine, the intern on duty Tuesday night, had run herself ragged on the ward, glancing down the long list of things that seemed to have been left undone the head nurse could only conclude that Jay Grossman, the assistant resident who had also been on call, had not done his share of the "scut work." There were numerous IVs that wanted restarting. Two of the leukemics already well into their poisons' course who had clearly needed platelets the night before had not gotten them. In 314, Mr. Solomon's leg was turning blue because a clot had cut off circulation. In 318, Mr. Alvarez, an alcoholic whose liver Dr. Newman had described yesterday as "about the size of a watermelon," had vomited a small amount of blood. In 322, one of the rooms for which Margaret Striker was personally responsible, Mrs. Volmer was down for an immediate transfer to the surgical ward to make way for a woman being transferred to 3H from coronary care, where, in turn, a bed was desperately needed for a man with a probable myocardial infarction who had been held in the emergency room for the last twelve hours. In 326, Jane Day's vital signs were erratic and her temperature showed a steady upward curve that might signal the end, and in 324, the head nurse's second room assignment, the embattled Mr. Blumenthal, who was still bleeding, needed a blood transfusion started before he could be given his Cryo today, and Walter Forsyth, the one person to whom Grossman had paid any real attention during the night, was evidently having difficulties too.

"What *did* Grossman do last night?" Margaret Striker asked Helen Fisk angrily as the two finished up changeover rounds. "Other than sleep?"

"He chased tail. There was a floater down at the other end, in 3G—a pretty new kid who didn't know Jay. He spent most of the night down there flirting with her. He's something else."

"Didn't Blaine get after him? I mean—four IVs infiltrated and not one restarted, and O'Hare not only *needed* platelets, she wasn't getting any Keflin. What if she spiked a fever and became septic while Grossman was chasing tail? Jesus Christ!" The head nurse cursed angrily.

"Blaine called him and called him and then she finally gave up and tried to do everything herself. But Jay did come back to see Forsyth and gave him his insulin at two."

"Did he say why he wanted to get him so tightly controlled? I don't even understand that. Mostly they want someone in his situation only loosely controlled when so much else might be going on. Did he stop the antibiotic?" she asked, momentarily forgetting Forsyth's orders from report and flipping through the card index for B side she carried in her arms to answer her own question as she and the night nurse made their way back to the nursing station.

"No, no," Helen Fisk answered her quickly. "He finishes up today."

"That's right," Margaret Striker responded. "They cultured up evidence of strep on Sunday in the lab work. But what the devil went on with him last night, Helen? He looks awful to me this morning—like he's in trouble with his electrolytes still. He's ashy pale, itchy, nervous, all upset about his lost baggage again. It could be the uncontrolled diabetes—sure—but with all that fluid at his ankles and the cloudy look in the urine, I'll bet his kidneys are messed up too." The head nurse paused thoughtfully, reviewing her reactions to Forsyth silently for any clues she might have missed. "Did Grossman happen to say anything revealing when he passed through last night to put in that Foley which maybe ought to come out?" she asked the LPN then. "Did he wonder about kidney function at all, or was he just his usual superior self?"

"Not much," the night nurse answered her. "But Kate Blaine told me Newman asked about creatinine clearances and all that stuff, as well as about his diabetic state. And I could see part of what was happening from the fracs. And then of course I got Marion Ping's report from the evening in detail."

Walter Forsyth's difficulties seemed to have begun almost immediately after Dr. Richards and Dr. Grossman had administered his first insulin injection just before supper the previous evening. Convinced that a low-grade strep infection which they were already treating with an oral antibiotic would minimize the effectiveness of the insulin, the two doctors pushed the usual experimental first dosage of the hormone up from twenty to forty units, justifying the move on the basis of yesterday's blood studies that had shown Forsyth's electrolyte balances to be mildly deranged, evidently as a result of his diabetes, a situation which indicated that he might possibly be progressing toward acidosis. But their boldness had produced disastrous results for Forsyth. Vomiting his supper, evidently in reaction to the insulin, he had spun into hypoglycemia—a state in which his blood-sugar levels were so low that the brain activities were impaired—and only speedy action by Marion Ring, who had recognized his situation on sight and forced him to drink sugared orange juice, had averted unconsciousness and possible insulin shock.

153

Yet despite Forsyth's demonstrated sensitivity to insulin, Dr. Grossman had evidently decided to pursue simultaneous control of his diabetes and developing acidosis by using glucose intravenously to keep the potassium levels in his plasma reduced while meantime covering its effects with injections of insulin every four hours while the nurses tracked the effectiveness of the regimen through hourly urine tests for excessive sugar. Catheterized so the nurses would not lose track of his urine output, Forsyth seemed to have done poorly, riding the metabolic roller coaster between sometimes dangerously high blood sugars and low ones as Grossman had continued to search for an insulin dosage that would cover his needs. This morning it was clear to the head nurse that each savage upward or downward swing had cost him some of his reserve and that Forsyth was drifting into some kind of trouble.

"I don't like any of it," Margaret Striker commented grimly after Helen Fisk finished her account of Forsyth's night. "There's nothing definite—nothing that diabetes coupled with an infection and a history like our friend's wouldn't explain. But I just feel spooked," she added, "like Grossman might be pushing him into something instead of keeping him out of it. I don't know," she sighed, realizing that until something definitive developed with Walter Forsyth she could not reasonably go to Steve Newman with her suspicions. "It's another game of wait and see, I guess. Wait and see on O'Hare too. Wait and see on Olsen. Wait and see on Blumenthal. Wait and see. Well." She was silent, running her eye down the problem list one more time. "Better scoot, Helen. I've already kept you too long. When did CCU want to send us their lady? Soon, I presume."

"Last night," Helen Fisk answered with a laugh. "And I said no way. But now it's as soon as you can get Mrs. Volmer out of here. You see, there's this guy with a heart attack down in the emergency room . . ." she began in an incredulous tone, shaking her head in disbelief.

"Yeah, yeah, yeah," said Margaret Striker, equally bemused. "But if he's not dead yet, after twelve hours with a developing MI he can go ten more minutes till I get Mrs. Volmer off this ward so CCU can send me their lady. What's her name, do you know?"

"George, I think," the black LPN responded, shrugging on her coat and preparing to go home. "Nancy George. They say she's a little strange—but in no present danger. I borrowed a monitor from G side for her."

As billed, Nancy George was " a little strange." Small and frail with bright blue eyes and flaring silver hair, she had a nervous avian quality and as she tried to assess her new environment while being wheeled onto 3H that morning her hands and eyes darted about in quick birdlike fashion. But Nancy George's anxiety was not, as the head nurse initially presumed, that of a typical cardiac patient afraid to leave the security of a small coronary care unit where she had felt constantly protected by ever watchful nurses. To the contrary, as Margaret Striker was later to learn, Miss George was relieved to be out of CCU, which she had perceived as some kind of strange laboratory, and was fearful of being moved onto 3H only because she was uncertain of where she was and why. Delusional in the wake of a massive heart attack, Miss George guessed that she was probably in St. Luke's, where she had been treated for Parkinson's disease some ten years before, and thought the year was probably 1964. With no apparent recollection of the searing pain in her chest that had brought her to the hospital eight days before, she was convinced that she had been felled in her fifteenth-floor apartment by "two men who flew in through her windows to rape and rob me."

"They wanted my heirlooms, you see," she explained earnestly to Margaret Striker as the head nurse was putting her to bed in 322, beginning to recount for the first time an improbable story she would repeat over and over again in the coming week. "They flew in the window to rob and rape me. Two men in black. Oh, I don't know what to do. My furniture was all I had left of my home. All my fortune," she said, frantically clutching the head nurse's wrist in her small, clawlike hand. Then, relaxing her fierce grasp, she had smiled beautifully and said persuasively,

"You're so good and kind, dear. Like the daughter I never had. I can see that I can trust you to help me. Call the police," she then whispered urgently. "Call the FBI."

When she had finished setting up a heart monitor in 322, where it appeared that Nancy George was going to be quite happy to be lodged with Caroline Blake, whose claim to be the Duchess of Windsor she evidently accepted without question, Margaret Striker returned to the nursing station to look at her chart and found Jay Grossman with his feet propped up on the desk already reading it.

"I see you've designated 322 as a wing of the psychiatric ward," the assistant resident said lightly, looking up from his reading. "Or did you put the two nuts together so they could share their similar interests?"

"Why do you say Miss George is a nut, Doctor?" the nurse said coolly, still thoroughly irritated with Jay Grossman for his sloppiness of the night before.

"Because it's all here," the assistant resident replied easily, tapping the aluminum cover of the chart that had accompanied Nancy George from coronary care. "Advanced arterial sclerosis, probable cardiac insufficiency following the MI, plus a history of Parkinson's. One more fruitcake, one more little old lady with senile dementia."

"Aren't you making up your mind a bit early?" the nurse said sharply. "You haven't even seen her yet. Couldn't the delusions be partly drug induced? Or do you make most of your medical judgments from the charts without seeing patients?"

"Most of 'em," the assistant resident said offhandedly, getting up and stretching, "because that's where the hard information is. In the charts and the lab work, not in my impressions of a patient's symptoms."

"Then what do your numbers tell you about Mr. Forsyth this morning, Dr. Grossman?" Margaret Striker inquired somewhat stiffly, her anger carefully controlled. "Because from where I stand —at the man's beside—he's sicker this morning than yesterday. His skin itches, he's irritable as the devil, and he feels rotten."

"They tell me," Jay Grossman answered in a mocking tone, "that I haven't gotten his diabetes under perfect control, which may explain why his electrolytes are still a little whacked up. But his BUN and creatinine clearances also tell me that there may be kidney involvement. It's that I intend to check out now. There was something vaguely shadowy about the left kidney on the admission X-rays, you see. Nothing definite, just something odd."

"Oh?" the head nurse responded, surprised to hear Jay Grossman confirm her own suspicion that a chronic kidney problem as much as uncontrolled diabetes lay at the root of Forsyth's present illness. "What do you propose to do about that?"

"Check the kidney," Grossman said flatly. "A retrograde pyelogram is scheduled for tomorrow."

"And Newman approves?" the nurse asked, startled because she knew that sometimes this test for kidney function could result in damage to the organ by allergic reactions to the dye or through impairment of the ureter, which, if both of Forsyth's kidneys were in a delicate state, could be particularly hazardous.

"Sure," Jay Grossman said with a shrug. "Why not? After all, Miss Striker, what I'm after is an explanation of his electrolyte troubles. We have to *know* if there's renal impairment, don't we? But don't worry your pretty little head about Mr. Forsyth," he continued. "Jay Grossman plays it safe. I go by the numbers in the lab tests and proofs from procedures. Right now it's my opinion that Forsyth is in no danger. But your Miss George *is* demented and will doubtless have to be placed in a state institution," he insisted, proffering Nancy George's chart. "Read it and weep."

Chapter 26

Margaret Striker had known Jay Grossman as an intern the previous year. She did not trust him. Big, with a square head and barrel chest mismatched with short arms and small hands, Grossman, despite a lumbering, bearlike appearance, not only considered himself sexually irresistible but was also intellectually vain. Cocky about his medical skills, the assistant resident tended to take chances his more cautious colleagues would avoid and, in the past, Margaret Striker had seen him push patients into trouble by overlooking important elements in a diagnosis enough times to make her believe that he might be mismanaging Walter Forsyth. But because no hard evidence of marginal kidney failure had yet emerged from the routine blood work either to dissuade Grossman from going through with the proposed pyelogram or to focus Steve Newman's attention on its possible danger to Forsyth, Margaret Striker found herself in the difficult position of trying to prod the assistant resident into considering the implied risks of the procedure by presenting him throughout Wednesday with the specific nursing observations that had given her reason to worry about the state of Forsyth's kidneys—namely, his elevated blood pressure, the pooling of fluid in his legs, his general irascibility, and the presence of traces of blood in his urine, all of which pointed to a chronic renal condition that might make this test hazardous if both kidneys were affected.

"Mr. Forsyth's blood pressure has been up there for several days, Jay," she remarked offhandedly to the assistant resident on finishing her morning rounds of the ward to collect vital signs. "He's 160 over 120 this morning and he's pretty cranky again today. . . .

"Say, Dr. Grossman, when I did the diabetic fractional on Mr. Forsyth's urine at ten there was a trace of blood in it.

"Forsyth has considerable edema at his ankles, Dr. Grossman. A bit worse than yesterday when I told you about it. I wonder if you want to take a look at him? I'm going to be in there with Dr. Blaine, helping to get Mr. Blumenthal's Cryo transfusion started," she told him at ten-thirty; after finishing her primary care in 324.

"By the way, Jay," she asked while picking up the morning orders at the nursing station at eleven, "did you get a chance to check Forsyth's edema? There really is quite a lot of fluid pooled in his ankles and feet. I've put him on strict intake and output records for today; I thought you'd want to keep careful track of his kidney function."

It was an exasperating situation for the head nurse, but not an unfamiliar one. In seven years in nursing Margaret Striker had lost most of her illusions professionally and become a realist in her relationship with doctors. She knew that just as there were nurses of all sorts—good, bad, and indifferent, concerned and callous—so were there all sorts of doctors, and none was flawless. As a fresh new surgical nurse she had learned this within her first month of hospital duty when, training in the operating room, she had seen a renowned surgeon accidently cut a coronary artery and kill his patient during a delicate open heart procedure, and the errors of commission and omission she had witnessed since had educated her to skepticism. Just as she knew no doctor was perfect, she knew no medical treatment was without attendant risk and no hospital's routines foolproof. To assume otherwise, especially on the busier wards in a big-city hospital like this one, was to be professionally naive to the point of irresponsibility and only increased the possibility of error. So despite the rules of hospital nursing that decreed that as a nurse Margaret Striker would defer to the physicians and follow orders unquestioningly, the head nurse did not hesitate to question the interns and residents on her ward whenever it seemed warranted for safety's sake.

But on 3H, as on all the other teaching units in this hospital, it was incidents like the present one involving Walter Forsyth that most perplexed and frustrated the nurses. While the best of the doctors generally were the most willing to listen to nurses' observations on their patients and the more cautious regularly sought comments from the head nurses, it seemed the rule that those doctors who most needed the nursing staff's help wanted it least and most resented their advice when it was given. And, to complicate the present situation, Margaret Striker knew that, unless she had indisputable proof that Jay Grossman's handling of Forsyth posed a potential threat to his patient's well-being to put before the chief resident, she was powerless to prevent the assistant resident from pursuing his plans for the man unless she could herself persuade Grossman to reconsider, or until his bungling became so apparent that Newman might be forced to intervene. Though the chief resident and even the senior physicians of the medical service might be willing to censure a junior member of the house staff for negligence after the fact, rarely were they inclined beforehand to reprimand them for being too aggressive with their patients even though in a teaching hospital like this one where many of the doctors were geared to believe in their own success and driven to prove themselves by accomplishment, by far the most common and cardinal of sins the physicians seemed to commit, from the nurses' point of view, was to push patients too far and exact answers on puzzling cases at a cost in risk and suffering that was far too high in human terms. But precisely because so many of the senior staff members were themselves medical "enthusiasts" and, in pursuit of knowledge, had themselves at one time or another been guilty of similar excesses, they seemed unwilling to curb the younger doctors and were offended when asked to do so by the nurses.

Initially the element of covert tyranny in the way certain doctors handled patients had infuriated Margaret Striker, but as she had rarely seen angry complaints from nursing to the senior house staff about such behavior produce satisfactory results, Margaret Striker had developed her own method for dealing with the Jay Grossmans of her world, and her favorite tactic was to play on their own vanity. By badgering them into worrying about how their handling of a case would appear to their colleagues she had discovered that she could usually force the careless to be careful and the callous to be more considerate. And so on Wednesday she had begun to play on Jay Grossman's fear of appearing foolish to Newman and the other doctors on 3H by harping most of the day on the possibility that he was mishandling Forsyth.

By midafternoon her tactics seemed to be paying off. Not only did the assistant resident adopt a number of suggestions from the head nurse which she believed might provide evidence that Forsyth was already in partial kidney failure, but before her afternoon books were closed except for emergency demands—Grossman had instructed that new blood samples be drawn on Forsyth for overnight lab analysis. Confident that if the blood report returned showing a progressive elevation in Forsyth's blood urea nitrogen, Grossman would consider the possibility his patient was in bilateral kidney failure and cancel the proposed test for fear manipulation might shut down Forsyth's left kidney or ureter and cause the right to be overloaded, Margaret Striker did not take her worries to Newman that evening even though Forsyth complained to her just before she left the floor that evening that he was "feeling queer."

"It's these stupid kid doctors," he had muttered when she and Stephanie Forester stopped at his bedside at four o'clock. "I gave 'em permission for some goddamned test they wanna do tomorrow when I was feeling okay earlier on, but now I'm not so sure I ought to go through with it. I need to talk the whole thing over with my son. I want you call him for me, Striker," he commanded gruffly, thrusting toward the head nurse a scrap of paper on which he had scribbled a New Jersey telephone number. "You're a good kid. Kind. I know you'll do this for me. Call him collect. Get him to come in here. Tell him there are certain papers I want to give him," he had added mysteriously, "papers he should have if anything happens to me."

"Nothing will happen to you," the head nurse had insisted firmly, giving Walter Forsyth a stock reply that did not betray her own lingering doubts. "If they decide to go through with the test tomorrow—and they may not—it'll be quite routine and perfectly safe," she had assured him. "So you've got nothing whatsoever to worry about."

But as she moved out of 324 into the corridor with Stephanie Forester after the two had stopped to speak with Harold Blumenthal, who was still anxiously waiting for word on the results of his midday transfusions of antihemophilic factor, she said in quite a different tone, "Watch Forsyth closely this evening, please, Stephanie. The intake and output records, up to the time you have to prep him for tomorrow—*if* you have to prep him—could be very important because if they turn up any more indications of progressive kidney failure Newman will be very much on guard in the morning and could cancel the test Grossman wants to do, especially if anything significant turns up in the lab this evening. My problem, however, is that so far nothing about Forsyth is conclusive. He's not oliguric—yet—so it's my hunch against Grossman's at this point, and you know how far I'd get taking an undocumented complaint to Newman. Grossman admits that Forsyth's in renal trouble, of course, or he wouldn't be doing a pyelogram. But he's looking for a tumor in the left kidney as the result of the sarcoma, and he's virtually disregarding the possibility that both kidneys may be infected or damaged independently of the cancer. He hasn't wanted to consider any of the signs Forsyth's been giving us all day of progressively worsening failure. I could be totally wrong, of course. It's obviously a very tricky case, but I just don't want to see him push Forsyth too far without even considering the guy's physical symptoms. I bet you Forsyth's kidneys are nephrotic and Jay's been using insulin and glucose to try to deal indirectly with his renal troubles. If he turned out to be sensitive to the dye and went into anaphylaxis or the ureter got blocked—bingo, that could do it for him. Newman's probably been all over Grossman about these possibilities at chart rounds, of course, but on the other side of it, Jay Grossman is not the kind of guy who really gives a damn about what's going on with his patients hour by hour. One test is enough for him—even though the lab results he goes on are hours old and evidence a patient is going sour is right before his eyes. So he could be telling Newman everything looks fine with Forsyth, while the guy's heading into shutdown. Maybe Forsyth *is* dying of cancer—but maybe he's got two more good years, and if he does I'd like to see he gets them, okay?" She paused then, standing outside of room 326, an expression of weariness on her face. "Now," she said quietly, "about Jane. She's febrile, but just keeps puffing along even though her diabetes is out of control. The policy is 'disinterested therapy.' No code 700. But I don't think anything will happen tonight. Her vital signs are steady. And Dela's okay too," she added with a wry smile. "If it's any consola-

162

tion to you, she was quite lucid today and talked about her grand-nieces."

"What's to become of her, Margaret?" Stephanie Forester asked, shaking her head slightly.

"I don't know," the head nurse replied. "Newman's starting to get itchy about getting her out of here—understandably. But the social worker hasn't found a workable placement yet, though one could come any day, so pray it does. . . ."

Chapter 27

The rains of autumn, brown in the dawn light, had come slamming down on the city the next morning with such ferocity that many months afterwards, when the year had come round again to fall, the sight of a similar equinoctial downpour would cause Margaret Striker to recall the final days of Steve Newman's tenure on 3H with the realization that her disenchantment with nursing even then had begun. But on that rainy Thursday, when she had reached the ward wet and cranky because she was late, she could not anticipate that events set in motion that day, which were to leave her feeling numb and somehow reduced, would mark the beginning of the end of her commitment to the head nurse's job so that when she resigned a year later to follow Eliot Cantor to Washington at his request, she would do so with a sense of relief.

But as she slumped into a chair in the dialysis room at five minutes after seven that morning, apologizing to the night nurse and the others for her lateness, what concerned Margaret Striker most was the question of how Mary Obakwanga would react to being disciplined. For as the head nurse had joined the others, the African RN, who had returned to work, responded to her arrival with a sullen look.

"You're half drowned, Miss Striker," Helen Fisk greeted her. "Don't you want to get a towel for your hair? I'm up to Mrs.

Suarez in 316A but since all our major troubles are concentrated on B side this morning, I don't think you've missed much."

"No, go ahead, Helen, please, I'll review the earlier stuff from the tape recorder and on changeover rounds with you later," the head nurse answered, shaking out her long, wet hair and pinning it up again.

"Okay then," the night nurse replied, picking up the card index and proceeding with her report on how the ward had fared from midnight until morning. "Mrs. Suarez in 316A. She's still clustering occasional PVCs but she's okay—on a monitor, resting comfortably with no complaint of chest pain. In B bed, Mrs. Olsen; we gave her Compazine at midnight and the Cytosine IV at two, with Thioguanine PO at the same time. Nothing to report on her except that she's getting very weak. Alvarez in 318, his ascites is way up . . . they're planning paracentesis today. . . ."

Fisk's voice droned on and the head nurse, picking up the vital signs, the significant oddities and details of the night nurse's report and filing them almost automatically in her mind, had taken the chance to study Mary Obakwanga as she listened. The African nurse had looked taut; there was a fidgety quality to her movements and twice when she had become aware of Margaret Striker's scrutiny she had turned her head to avert the head nurse's gaze with an angry look.

"In 322, Mrs. Blake had a very royal evening but Miss George in B bed slept right through it!" Fisk was saying, beginning to wind up her report. "Miss George is on a monitor, she's okay—in normal sinus rhythm except for slight atrial flutter occasionally. In 324, Mr. Blumenthal got a three per cent gain in circulating AHF following yesterday's eleven thousand units of Cryo, but though he didn't bleed in the night, Dr. Blaine told Stephanie Forester last night that she didn't expect the gain to hold up for long. In B bed, Mr. Forsyth. He complained of headache last night and his blood pressure is 150 over 116. He is prepped for a pyelogram this morning."

"He's what?" Margaret Striker interrupted her in surprise.

"Didn't Newman cancel that last evening? Didn't Forester say anything about his last blood report?"

"Nobody told me nothing, Miss Striker, except he was going for the kidney test this morning at nine," Helen Fisk answered her. "Forester prepped him and I was in and out of there last night a lot and nobody told him anything different about today either. Why?"

"Oh, I guess it's me," Margaret Striker answered. "I would have sworn the guy was in partial kidney failure, but if the lab work didn't show his blood urea nitrogen was elevated, well, evidently I was overreacting. . . ."

"Well," Helen Fisk responded thoughtfully, "I'd have said the same thing 'bout him last night. He was kinda sick, you know, sweaty, itchy, jumpy. And Forester said when his son came by he was awful agitated too. But I guess if the tests were ordered the doctors think he'll tolerate it okay. His intake and output records are charted, if you wanna take a look."

"No—you're right, of course. If they think he can tolerate it, I've probably just exaggerated his symptoms in my own mind," Margaret Striker answered. "Go on, Helen, excuse the interruption."

"In 326," the night nurse continued, "Mrs. Hanze slept through the night. Hallelujah! Not a peep or a honk. But in B bed, Jane Day's not good. Dr. Cantor was on last night and he's in with her now. He thinks it's maybe another CVA evolving. He asked that you join him in there when you could, Miss Striker. He paged Dr. Fischer earlier on, but couldn't rouse him—probably at breakfast. In C bed, Mrs. O'Brien's temperature is coming down; she's at 100.4 so they think she's responding well to the antibiotic; she's on gentomycin with an IV to KVO. In D bed, Mrs. Franklin—they say she'll go home tomorrow. . . ."

After she had made changeover rounds with Helen Fisk and told Mary Obakwanga that she wanted a conference with her at ten, Margaret Striker made her way to 326, where she found Eliot Cantor, who had drawn the curtains around B bed, standing inside of the shadowy confines of the cloth cubicle they formed, watching Jane Day's irregular breathing.

"How is she, Eliot?" the head nurse had asked softly as she stepped into the twilight beside him. "What are her vital signs?"

"She's expiring, I think," the intern said simply in a subdued tone, swiftly providing the nurse with the pertinent figures on pulse, blood pressure, and respiration. "Respiratory disruptions all the time now. I think it's cerebral infarction. There have been some convulsions. I couldn't raise Fischer with a page at six-thirty after this started. I just want to be certain about not calling a code on her. Will you stay here while I phone Newman?" he asked, his gentle face smudged below the eyes with shadows of exhaustion, pale in the gloom. "I'd just feel better if I told him how she was dying and confirmed that we shouldn't attempt to resuscitate."

"Sure, Eliot," the nurse said simply, aware of how contrary to the intern's training it was not to act to prevent life slipping away. "Go phone Steve and take your time about it," she said, certain herself that any attempt to save Jane Day was pointless. "I'll wait with Jane."

When death came, it came quietly, the dim, flickering tensions of life fading gradually from the big, work-worn body like a brightness dimming in some shadowed light-patterned place to be missed only after it is gone. "There should have been a sound of bells or oboes, some sad song from somewhere for Jane," Margaret Striker thought absently as she had watched the singular tautness of vitality fade, but instead there was only the sounds from the rain-swept avenue outside, of traffic swishing interminably by and quarrelsome horns in leit motif. Death's music, instead, was a silence in the cubicle, the absence of the sound of Jane Day's breathing as the tautness of her body broke and it lay slack-limbed and uninhabited on the rumpled sheets of the bed, the calloused skin of the big black hands too relaxed in death, sloughing whitely away.

Yet as Margaret Striker drew a sheet over her face and stood alone for a moment in the lilac gloom of the cubicle she felt relieved rather than regretful that Jane Day was gone. In the two and a half months that she had lain in this bed more than forty-five thousand dollars, charged to Medicaid, had been expended on caring for her, a sum that Jane Day, a retired domestic, would never have seen in a lifetime of cleaning other people's apartments. But what had been prolonged had not been Jane Day's life, but her dying.

"Jane's gone, Eliot," she told the intern, whom she met returning to 326 as she headed toward the nursing station to report the death. "At seven fifty-six exactly. She was Cheyne-Stoking and then she just stopped breathing for the last time and didn't start again. I checked the pulses. They were extremely thready and erratic and then it was over. I didn't try to restart the heart."

"I'm sorry, Margaret," the intern said, turning to walk beside her toward the nursing station, giving her shoulder a comforting pat. "I should have been with you. But you did the right thing. Newman confirmed we weren't to resuscitate."

"Poor old Jane," the assistant head nurse responded simply when Margaret Striker told her of the death. "But there's other bad news too. Obakwanga has resigned; came in late yesterday and gave her notice. Nancy Maxwell called while you were in 326. She hasn't told anybody here yet—as far as I can see. I think she's saving it for you. Nancy says not to worry. She'll get us a replacement if she has to kidnap an RN from New York Hospital."

"Mm? Thanks," Margaret Striker replied, still so distracted by Jane Day's passing that she hardly responded to the problem of staffing implied by Marie Velasquez's news. "You know, Marie, you never really get over it," she said suddenly, speaking from her emotions for a moment. "You gear yourself for it. Tell yourself you're used to it and in a case like Jane's, rationally, you even wish for it for weeks. But when it comes, and you stand there and do nothing, it takes something out of you, you know? A little chip of you goes every time. . . ."

"Every time, kid," Marie Velasquez answered, sympathetically lingering at the nursing station. "Though I think what they finally did with Jane was the right thing. It should have happened a while back—you know it and I know it. It's just the emptiness you feel afterwards that gets to you and leaves a lot of unshed tears."

"Do you know what Nancy told me about the new kids?" Margaret Striker replied. "Some are being told during training that it's all right to cry with and for your patients. That sharing grief has a real place in nursing. Isn't that a good thing, Marie? Too bad it comes a little late for old horses like us. Leaves us with all this gunk bottled up inside. Wears you out, huh?"

"I don't know," Marie Velasquez answered. "When I started, I cried all the time. Took everything home with me. Now I leave it here most of the time and only cry once in a while. In crazy, unexpected places, when I see something like my kids being happy. And at the movies. Boy, do I cry at the movies. My husband takes four handkerchiefs with him every time we go to a sad movie. Not Kleenex—I pulverize Kleenex. Handkerchiefs. It's my thing, I guess." She paused, waiting to see if the head nurse needed to talk about Jane Day further before she remarked simply, "Look, Margaret, I don't really know anymore which is best, being involved or keeping it cool. But I do know this—unless you have a way to hang on to your own heart, you use yourself up, piece by piece, parcel by parcel, until there's no more to give. Some nurses can take from their patients and that keeps them strong. Me, I take from my family *and* my patients. But you? You just give and drive and push and don't take back much, and, Margaret, you need to, 'cause you're knocking yourself out in this job already. Trying so hard to make up for all the screw-ups, the doctors who don't give a damn, the lazy people. Cool it a little, Margaret. Ease up. Take something back from what you give. You'll last longer."

The head nurse, leaning on the desk, a bruised look in her dark blue eyes, nodded almost imperceptibly in response and then began dialing Central Records to report Jane Day's death. "I can't ease up, Marie," she said quietly. "I don't think I know how."

Chapter 28

"Ease up," Marie Velasquez had said. "Don't push." But when Margaret Striker glanced at the time after notifying the hospital authorities that Jane Day had died, she found that she was already half an hour behind a schedule she had set for herself and that the clock had quietly, mechanically destroyed her chance for a lengthy round of the ward that morning. She had wanted to see several patients whom she had been forced to neglect during Mary Obakwanga's two-day absence from the floor—especially Tanya Olsen, Nancy George, Harold Blumenthal, and Mary O'Malley, all of whom were as besieged emotionally as they were physically. But as she calculated the time left to her to check IVs, monitors, and staff work in order to be back at the nursing station to speak to Steve Newman before he began his morning rounds, Margaret Striker realized she would have less than ten minutes to spare for visiting with patients and chose to use them talking with Mary O'Malley.

Mark Eaglesbury had given her a worrisome report Wednesday on the young stewardess. Though understandably disturbed and frightened by the news that the lymphangiogram had located sites of malignancy in her abdomen as well as chest so that she had been classified as having stage IIB Hodgkin's disease, Mary O'Malley had not as yet consented to be treated and the intern, baffled and outraged by what seemed to him willful madness on the girl's part, had complained to Margaret Striker that he thought one of her nurses, Janet St. Clair, might be partly responsible for the stewardess's refusal to accept therapy immediately. "St. Clair's been meddling," Eaglesbury had warned the head nurse stiffly. "I don't understand what her hold over the girl is, but if she weren't in the picture we'd have had permission to begin treatment the day we staged her. . . ."

But when Margaret Striker had questioned Janet St. Clair about Mary O'Malley's motives for declining help on Wednesday afternoon, she had been more mystified than enlightened by the nurse's response.

"She needs time," Janet St. Clair had said. "She shouldn't be pushed into intensive irradiation. She wants to think—think about her options, about her life. . . ."

"What's to think about?" Margaret Striker had asked, bewildered. "Does she understand that with treatment she can have five, ten, maybe even fifteen more years of life, but that without it she may be dead in two years?"

"She understands," the nurse had answered with a curiously tight expression. "But she wants to think about how to use those years—as many as there may be."

"What do you mean, Janet?" Margaret Striker had asked, as distressed by the look that had come into Janet St. Clair's face then as she was by her response. "What possible reason could a twenty-six-year-old woman have for throwing her life away?"

"She has her reasons for what she's doing," Janet St. Clair had responded cryptically. "Reasons I'm afraid I understand too well," the nurse had continued. "But maybe I'm too close to this. Maybe you should talk to her—help her sort it all out," Janet St. Clair had added. "Ask her why, Margaret. Tell her we talked."

Yet on Thursday morning as Margaret Striker approached Mary O'Malley, whom she found standing at the end of the corridor staring from the rain-smeared window down to the storm-battered streets, the head nurse hesitated, glancing at her watch. "Ten minutes isn't enough time to ask anybody about dying." The head nurse later remembered thinking with a bleak sense of the absurdity of her mission, when, in the look Mary O'Malley gave her as she turned her head from the window she had recognized panic and vulnerability. "Better to be silent," she thought vaguely. "Better simply to stand next to this girl, who is my own age, and say nothing at all." "I know why you've come, Miss Striker," Mary O'Malley greeted her in a small voice, her southern drawl evident in the way she pronounced the head nurse's name. "But, you see, this is something that Dr. Eaglesbury simply can't understand."

"What doesn't he understand, Mary?" Margaret Striker asked her quietly, touched by the girl's youth and her pale frailty and not wanting to see the look of entrapment in her gray eyes. "He has told me you are refusing treatment for reasons he cannot fathom."

"No, no, not refusing," Mary O'Malley answered quickly. "It's just that I need time. Hasn't Janet explained to you why?"

"We have talked," the head nurse answered, offering no further comments.

"Then you know about Janet," Mary O'Malley said in almost a whisper. "So you *must* understand about me. Except that perhaps you don't know about my son. . . ."

Briefly and apparently without emotion Mary O'Malley told Margaret Striker her story. Born in Texas, she had grown up in one of the suburban communities scattered along the bayous of Galveston Bay and after high school she had gone to work in Houston as an airlines ticket clerk.

Ambitious, she had eventually won the chance to train as a stewardess. "I had a way out of Texas then," she said softly. "A ticket to someplace. The life was exciting. Everybody lived easy. Here one day, someplace else the next. San Francisco was my favorite town. I was crazy about it." She had fallen in love with a pilot in San Francisco. He was married. She had become pregnant. Hoping to persuade him to divorce his wife, she had refused to have an abortion. The baby, a boy, had been born in San Francisco the previous May, but by then the affair had ended. She had put her son up for adoption and gone back to work for another airline. Early in the summer she had begun to feel peculiar. Three months later she had been diagnosed as having Hodgkin's disease and sent to this hospital for "staging." By then she was based in New York, flying in and out of Kennedy Airport on the runs to the South. "I was still new in town when I got sick. Nobody here in New York really knows me," she told Margaret Striker quietly. "Oh, I have a few girl friends, other stewardesses, but they come and go—we are seldom together for any time at all. It's a funny life, really. You have hotel rooms or apartments, suitcases here, clothes there, but no place is home and no friend's

171

steady. . . . Well—there was nobody I could talk to really when I learned how sick I might be, nobody to cry with or tell about my son. And all of a sudden New York scared me. I was caught in something that seemed to be chopping me up—but if I yelled, nobody would really hear me, do you know what I mean?" She hesitated, her gray eyes searching Margaret Striker's face. "So I suppose that's why I told Janet everything right off, even before I knew how far along my disease was. Somehow I felt she understood instinctively what I was going through even before she told me she had Hodgkin's too."

Margaret Striker, concentrating on Mary O'Malley's words, did not react. Below her on the avenue, a woman carrying a red umbrella who was running for a bus narrowly missed being struck by a taxi that had swerved suddenly and unpredictably out of the line of traffic. "That's how it happens," Margaret Striker said to herself in a whisper. "It comes obliquely." As she spoke, in her mind's eye she saw the agonized face of a dark-haired woman lying in a bed, the first patient whom she had nursed in surgical metabolism and let die so many years ago. "Hit by a taxi," the doctors had explained when they brought the woman with one leg to the unit. "Really smashed her up." Margaret Striker wondered how many thousand people she had watched die in the lifetime that seemed to have passed since then. "Death comes randomly, doesn't it?" the head nurse murmured, startling Mary O'Malley.

"What? What did you say, Miss Striker?" the girl responded.

"Clip, bang. That lady down there with the red umbrella could have been killed," Margaret Striker replied, thinking, "Mary is twenty-six. Janet is twenty-six. I am twenty-six. Why them and not me?"

That morning, Jane Day's death had seemed, at last, natural and fitting. But too many others seemed to die as a matter of happenstance. They stood on the wrong corners. They got the wrong genes, like Harold Blumenthal, who would one day bleed to death. A random selection produced a protocol for the treatment of leukemia that was practically as lethal as the disease itself. Or

172

maybe something went askew in the immune system and at twenty-six suddenly you had to consider how few years of life might be left to you and ask yourself how to use them. Margaret Striker looked at her watch then. She would be late for Steve Newman. It was getting on toward nine. She must make rounds still. "You will find your routines are sound—stay with them and when you're in trouble, lean on them," she remembered some instructor telling her class in nursing school. "Don't push," Marie Velasquez had said, "hang on to your own heart."

"So now perhaps you understand," Mary O'Malley was saying. "It's not that I'm refusing treatment altogether. Dr. Eaglesbury just doesn't understand. It's that I have to find *myself* somehow. Put my life together. Right now I feel like I'm hooked into a computer or something, you know? I'm programmed for a flight to Atlanta and then on to Dallas with radiation therapy on Thursdays. It doesn't make sense—any of it. I don't want to die, but I can't stay here and have them burn away part of my life either. I have to go home. I have to try to reclaim my son if I can and go home to live where people know me and I know them so I can watch my son start to grow up where, if I have to leave him again, people will know he was mine. So now you see, Miss Striker, why I won't give the doctors my consent. It's that I have to leave something of myself whole, just like Janet. If I can find my son— take him back to Texas—then I'll go up to Houston for radiation treatment, I promise you. But if I've lost him—well, maybe I *want* to take a chance. Maybe I can get by the way Janet has. It's three years since they diagnosed her as the same stage of Hodgkin's I am, Hodgkin's two B. Sounds like a course at the New School, doesn't it? But, you see, she's hung on even though she wouldn't let them use X-ray on her abdomen. Her chest, yes, but not over her womb and ovaries, and she still hopes to have a baby one day. She fought them for that and went on to chemotherapy and got a remission. And she's still okay. I think she's incredibly brave, don't you? But because of her, I'm determined to try the same thing, if I can. . . ."

Below, on the street, the woman with the red umbrella had retreated to the safety of the sidewalk, where she stood waiting for a bus to detach itself from the stream of traffic and come to the curb.

"You do understand, Mary," Margaret Striker asked Mary O'Malley soberly, "that your prognosis with treatment may be excellent?"

"I do," Mary O'Malley answered in a whisper.

"And you do understand that if you get a full remission from your disease now, advances in treatment may possibly arrive at a cure before you would need further treatment with chemotherapy?"

Mary O'Malley nodded. "I have to go home, Miss Striker," she said very quietly. "Tell Dr. Eaglesbury I just have to go home."

Below them, the woman with the red umbrella boarded a bus which disappeared up the avenue and the tenuous thread that had for a few moments connected her life to the lives of the two young women who stood at the window on 3H was broken.

Chapter 29

Stunned by the news about Janet St. Clair, Margaret Striker began making her rounds of the ward almost mechanically but as she moved from room to room to find that in 312 the wall outlet for oxygen had again broken down, that in 316 Tanya Olsen, who had been scheduled to receive a blood transfusion on Wednesday evening, had not yet gotten it, that Mrs. Suarez's monitor was malfunctioning, that breakfast trays had not been distributed to some patients, and that for the second time in a week the interns had neglected patients whose IVs were painfully infiltrated, the head nurse's first reaction of pity for Janet St. Clair was overlaid by something near desperation. For if Mary O'Malley's account of her situation had proven accurate, not only was Janet St. Clair's personal prognosis uncertain, but the news about her in effect meant that Margaret Striker had probably lost not one but two nurses that morning. To move from radiation to chemotherapy in the treatment of Hodgkin's disease usually indicated that the malignancy had multiple locations in the lymph system, and if this were true it seemed possible that Janet St. Clair might only be in partial remission. If so, before very long she would need to be rehospitalized for another round of chemotherapy and since she had come close to admitting her state to Margaret Striker on Wednesday, the head nurse thought that the time might now be close at hand—a probability that she found dispiriting both personally and professionally. For with Mary Obakwanga leaving in a matter of weeks and Janet St. Clair perhaps within the month, how, Margaret Striker had wondered, would she manage to keep the ward running decently? It was a question that she would ask herself repeatedly throughout the day. Thursday, as events began crowding one upon the other until, when four o'clock came, it seemed impossible that the day that had ended with Walter Forsyth becoming feverish had begun with Jane Day's death.

The pressure on Margaret Striker had mounted steadily from the moment she returned to the nursing station just after nine to find herself too late to see the chief resident before he made rounds of the ward. First there had been a quarrel with the clerk in the blood bank about the lost blood order for Tanya Olsen. Then a phone call had come from the social worker, asking the head nurse to fill out another set of papers for Dela Hanze immediately and have them signed by the doctors that morning to take advantage of an unexpected opportunity to place Mrs. Hanze in a reputable nursing home within the week. At ten the meeting with Mary Obakwanga, though anticlimactic, had nevertheless proven to be a strain as the African nurse had unleashed her resentments and frustrations on Margaret Striker. These extra demands on her time, overlaid on her usual tightly scheduled routine, were precisely the kind that she feared would receive short shrift if her staff were further reduced and she had to take on staff nursing responsibilities herself. At ten-thirty Darlene Blumenthal appeared unexpectedly at the nursing station, having maneuvered her way past the security guards that kept visitors off the wards until the afternoon. Drawn and frightened, she had driven in from New Jersey through the storm, seized by the conviction that her husband was dying and once again the time and emotional energy required to reassure her had tightened Margaret Striker's schedule. It was eleven o'clock before she could begin picking up orders and badgering the doctors for renewals, yet comforting Mrs. Blumenthal, dealing with staff problems, grappling with bureaucracy to keep Mrs. Hanze from being maltreated, squabbling with the system to be sure that Tanya Olsen got blood, all "irregular" activities, were nevertheless essential aspects of Margaret Striker's job, not simply because they were part of her duty but because in putting things right for patients when they went wrong and in her small triumphs over the "system's" indifference, Margaret Striker found a special satisfaction. "Keeping it human," she called it, "fighting off the machine and keeping the place human." But comforting griefs and untying bureaucratic tangles was an unending business and that morning just after she had seen Darlene Blumenthal off the floor, a new wrangle with Jay Grossman erupted over Nancy George.

Since Miss George had been sent to 3H from the coronary care unit, Jay Grossman had been insisting that, like her roommate, Caroline Blake, whom the staff referred to as the Duchess, Nancy George was suffering from an irreversible senile dementia and he had been agitating for a "psych consult" in order to set in motion the machinery for having both women discharged to state mental institutions. It was a move Margaret Striker did not support both because she was convinced that some of Miss George's confusions were attributable to drugs she had been receiving and would soon abate, and because things she had been told by some of Miss George's visitors had made the head nurse suspect that there might be a rational foundation even for Miss George's outrageous story that two men had flown in through her windows to attack her which needed to be checked before the addled woman was subjected to a psychiatric interview.

According to Miss George's friends, her apartment was, as claimed, almost entirely though sparsely furnished with valuable antiques, heirlooms Nancy George had inherited. The last of a once wealthy southern family, Miss George had come to New York in the 1920s and through social connections she had set herself up in the business of placing the daughters of the "gentry" in careers in keeping with their debutante standing. Her placement agency, which had handled only the white-gloved nieces of Park Avenue clients for years, had proven so successful that, though admittedly no longer wealthy herself, Nancy George had moved easily in rarified social circles even after the 1929 stock market crash, and until well into the 1950s, having earned a blueblood reputation, her placement agency had thrived. When Nancy George had retired, she had seemed secure. But then, a variation of Parkinson's disease, the belated sequel to an encephalitis misdiagnosed as influenza during the epidemic of the 1920s, had struck her. She had spent months in St. Luke's Hospital in 1963 before being returned home, palsied, but with the Parkinson's stabilized. In this period she had used up most of her savings to pay her medical bills and since 1963 had supported herself in part by the sale of her antiques. Her friends had explained to Margaret Striker that recently Miss George's precarious financial state had begun to terrify her.

On the evening of her heart attack Miss George had invited a friend to tea. When the woman arrived and rang the bell she thought she heard a stunned shout and then something fall inside Miss George's apartment, but when her hostess did not answer her doorbell the friend had left. She had begun calling a little later, telephoning the apartment every half hour until after six o'clock. Then, convinced that Miss George was in trouble, she had called the police, who had somehow entered the locked apartment to find Nancy George unconscious and had brought her to the hospital.

Treated for myocardial infarction—death of part of the heart muscle as a result of blockage of blood flow through one of the tiny coronary arteries—Miss George had been kept in the coronary care unit for a week under constant sedation and then was transferred to 3H. When she had arrived on the unit she was still showing the full-blown effects both of her MI and of the drugs used to treat it—disorientation, confusion, and even amnesia—all of which Margaret Striker, as a former coronary care nurse, knew might yet clear if Miss George was given time.

But by Thursday noon, time appeared to be running out for Miss George. Arguing that cardiac insufficiency and long-term arterial disease had resulted in considerable damage to Miss George's brain, Jay Grossman had evidently persuaded Steve Newman to have the psychiatrists consider Nancy George for possible placement in a mental institution. Though Margaret Striker knew that there were checks against anyone being placed in a state hospital without sufficient cause, if she was to protect Miss George from the strain of a group psychiatric examination, which would be conducted as much to teach the interns and residents how to interview such a patient in psychiatric terms as to determine the truth about Nancy George's mental state, it seemed imperative that the head nurse discover just how the police had made entry to Nancy George's locked apartment.

She began by calling the emergency room to find out if anyone there remembered Miss George; no one did. Next she attempted to make contact through the precinct headquarters with the unknown policemen who had responded to the call from Nancy George's friend, and finally, at two o'clock, one of the officers actually returned her repeated calls.

When the alarm about Miss George had come in, he told Margaret Striker, he and a partner had been dispatched in their patrol car to her address. Finding her apartment locked, and unable to break down the metal door, they had finally entered it by crawling along an outside ledge from an adjacent apartment and had broken in through the windows to rescue Miss George, whom they found lying on her living room floor. Semiconscious at the time, Miss George had evidently seen them as they crashed through the glass—two men in black, apparently flying into her fifteenth-floor apartment through the windows to attack her.

When Margaret Striker told Steve Newman the policeman's story of rescuing Nancy George, the chief resident was persuaded that in view of the circumstances surrounding her heart attack and her generally anxious state prior to the infarction, it was possible that Miss George's "delusions" were less serious than they appeared. The "psych-consult" in which Jay Grossman would have "presented" Nancy George as a study in senile dementia was canceled and after asking Margaret Striker to notify the social service department about her, Newman indicated that he would recommend having Miss George temporarily placed in an extended care facility where her Medicare benefits would cover most of her costs until her true mental state could be determined.

Added to the other small victories, this one would have left Margaret Striker feeling well pleased with the day despite the harassments and worries it had brought her if she had not been forced to report to Newman in the same conversation that Walter Forsyth had become febrile. The nurses had found that he was running a temperature of 101 during a routine check on vital signs, and though Margaret Striker had no definite reason to suspect a connection between this symptom of renewed infection somewhere in Forsyth's body and the pyelogram that had been performed this morning, she was nevertheless unnerved by the coincidence. For if her original suspicions about Walter Forsyth proved true and a chronic kidney ailment had left him with both kidneys weakened, she knew that this fever might indicate that the pyelogram, which had been done by pushing radioactive dye from Forsyth's bladder back into the left kidney with a catheter, had exacerbated a pre-existing condition and could signal the beginning of a crisis. And when the head nurse considered Dr. Newman's reaction to her report about Nancy George, she could not but wonder if by having failed to take her worries about Walter Forsyth to the chief resident on Wednesday she had not been danerously derelict in her duty to him.

Chapter 30

Climbing onto the bus the next morning, the storm-washed sky of dawn silver with tattered clouds blown in from the restless spaces of the sea, Margaret Striker found herself dealing death to her fellow passengers, finding in the muddled, contradictory look of age in this face the stamp of vascular disease and in that yellowed eye the certainty of jaundice. After ten hours in bed she was still tired, for her sleep had been plagued by nightmares and her waking by worries left over from the previous day. She felt numb and angry, for almost by accident just before going home on Thursday she had learned that Jay Grossman had apparently disregarded all of her warnings about Walter Forsyth and, despite the evidence that both of his kidneys might be weakened by chronic infection, had subjected him to a pyelogram on the basis of blood work already twenty-four hours old when Forsyth went to X-ray without so much as taking the precaution of testing him beforehand for a possible reaction to the dye.

It had all emerged when the head nurse had met Dr. Richards at the elevators the previous evening as she was leaving the floor and talked with him about Walter Forsyth.

"Your man in 324 is febrile, Frank," she had told the intern tiredly, jabbing the down button. "I've informed Newman because I couldn't find either you or Grossman on the floor. There's a nursing note from me in his chart and I've posted vital signs. I must say I'm concerned about him; I thought yesterday he looked nephritic. How'd the pyelogram go this morning anyway?"

"He was bad for a bit," Richards had answered, surprising her. "Seemed to go sour right before our eyes and then come back out of it again. For a second he scared me. I was afraid of anaphylactic shock," the intern had admitted, referring to an exaggerated allergenic reaction to the dye used in pyelography which, though not common, nevertheless could occur as a side-effect of the test and result in death. "He had all signs, you know."

"But he wasn't allergic to the dye, was he?" the nurse had asked, letting a down elevator go by without her. "What did the sensitivity tests show?"

"We didn't do any sensitivity tests," Richards had replied, not meeting her eyes. "They aren't done routinely, and in his case they didn't seem necessary; he has no history of allergies. So I cannot really say whether he was allergic or not. But the danger of anaphylaxis is past now, and in any case we've other fish to fry with him now. Question is, of course, what state his right kidney is in if by any chance we get a problem with his left kidney as a result of manipulation. He's been slightly acidotic, as you know," the intern had continued, gaining confidence as he spoke and unaware of the effect of his words on the nurse. "What we have here is a case of sarcoma—evidently in remission—overlaid by diabetes and more recently by a fever of still unknown origin," Dr. Richards had gone on, lecturing the nurse much as if he were addressing an auditorium full of physicians. "Hence, the reasons for acidosis are multiple. With the pyelogram, we were looking for specific renal damage, and though I haven't reviewed the film myself I'm certain we'll find a tumorous mass in the left kidney even though yesterday his electrolytes were not particularly disturbed. But there were hints in the morning creatinine clearances and in the BUN that he might be in slight failure and . . ."

"What did the six-channel blood test from last night show?" the nurse had interrupted him, suddenly uneasy. "He wasn't acidotic then, was he?"

"The evening bloods?" Richards had answered defensively. "Oh —the lab lost those. . . ."

Shaken, Margaret Striker had stepped into the down elevator that opened its doors at that moment without another word to Dr. Richards, for what she had just heard not only meant that Jay Grossman had given no weight to her nursing observations in his decision to send Forsyth for the pyelogram but that her suspicion that she had failed in her duty as a head nurse when she had not taken her concerns about Forsyth to Newman had been confirmed. Yet though the anger, frustration, and guilt she had felt in that moment were with her still the next morning, her mood as she stepped off the elevator onto 3H on Friday was less one of indignation than acquiescence. For it now seemed almost inevitable to her that what had happened to Walter Forsyth had had to happen—that like the city it served, the hospital, as a product of supreme technology, was at times possessed by forces that had lost all sense of human scale, and that in its absorption with its own wizardry it had become an institution bound to produce among its doctors soulless technicians like Jay Grossman, whose arrogance and absorption with demonstrable "results" made them careless of individuals. And as she walked wearily toward the nursing station that morning Margaret Striker was as certain that in the future there would be other Forsyths on 3H as she was that there would be other Dr. Grossmans and that she would always be too harried to prevent the kind of bungling indifference that had perhaps already pushed Walter Forsyth to the point of no return. The head nurse's job, she now realized, was too diffuse, too demanding. Expected to keep medicine "humane" by seeing that the patients' needs were met, there was always too much detail, too much paperwork, and too many problems to be seen to for anyone to perform faultlessly in the role, though anything less than perfect performance, she knew, could result in harm to patients both physically and spiritually, as it had with Forsyth. The trick, it was beginning to seem, was to accept this without despairing—to learn to tolerate the intolerable.

"How's Forsyth?" she asked Helen Fisk before going to her locker to put away her coat. "Anything new on him?"

"What are you, a seer?" the night nurse asked, raising her eyebrow. "Yeah, man, he's in trouble. Up and down on the fracs, up and down on the fever all night, and he's been half stuporous or crazy a lot of the time. He'd sleep and then wake up shoutin' 'bout his papers, 'bout going home, 'bout getting his son in here. Even yelled for you coupla times. Eaglesbury says its his electrolytes. That six-channel Grossman sent out on Wednesday finally turned

up last night. He was bad even before that pyelogram, Eaglesbury told me, but I didn't need no lab tests to tell me what I
could see with my eyes, Miss Striker. That poor man was sick the
night before last, no question, and sicker still last night. His blood
pressure up at 190 over 130 now, and when I did my last rounds
on vital signs, when I was checking his pulse it felt kinky, you
know? I listened to his heartbeat and he was throwin' arrhythmias
then. But I been watching him close since and nothin' else
showed so I didn't wake the doctors. I mean—you know how teed
off they get. . . ."

Pulling Forsyth's chart from the rack before she went to report,
Margaret Striker looked up the second six-channel blood report on
him that was dated September 18. The figures in it confirmed
Fisk's assessment and her own worst suspicions. Even before the
pyelogram had been done, there had been evidence Forsyth was
in partial renal failure. Though his sodium levels on Wednesday
had been in the normal range, the other electrolytes were charted
in a pattern that reminded the head nurse of a city skyline. His
potassium levels had been too high at 6.3, his carbon dioxide had
been depressed, his blood urea nitrogen had been up at 115, and
his glucose elevated to 230. It was a profile of electrolyte imbalances which begged for caution in dealing with Walter Forsyth's
kidneys that Jay Grossman had not shown. Now, it appeared
likely that added to the damaging impact of infection and diabetes
on his kidneys, the dehydration brought about by prepping him
for the pyelogram and the effects of manipulation during the test
had exacerbated a pre-existing kidney problem, driving Forsyth
into hazardous straits in which his electrolytes were dangerously
deranged. The pulse irregularity Helen Fisk had reported pointed
to the possibility that the potassium in Forsyth's bloodstream had
already reached toxic levels and this alarmed the head nurse sufficiently to send her in search of Bill Fischer, the assistant resident
on duty, immediately. If Walter Forsyth went into renal shutdown
and, as a result, the poisons in his bloodstream battered his heart
to a standstill, the head nurse knew she would not be able to es-

scape a share in the guilt for the bungling that had brought him so close to death.

The head nurse found Dr. Fischer asleep in the conference room and wakened him with her report on Forsyth. Dismayed, the blue-eyed assistant resident shook his head slowly. "What time is it?" he asked sleepily. "Won't Grossman be coming on soon? The guy is his patient, after all, so I don't want to start aggressive therapy if I haven't got to right away. Jeez," he mumbled quietly, pausing to think. "But yeah—get an ECG set up so we know where he's at," he said then, nodding. "I'll be right there. If he's way wide I'll probably start kayexelate right away and try to knock down the potassium. And get Mark to draw bloods on him stat too, okay? Whatever happens, Newman's gonna want those when he gets here no matter what we do."

He rose, reaching for a strawberry-colored shirt he had hung over the back of the chair as Margaret Striker closed the door and went to wake Mark Eaglesbury, who was sleeping in the patient lounge, before she began setting up an ECG machine in Forsyth's cubicle. In testing it she pulled a single rhythm strip on the first lead and took a quick look at it. Though only moderately distorted, the pattern of Forsyth's heartbeat, showing wide, tent-shaped T-waves, seemed to her eye to indicate that he was already carrying an excessive potassium load in his bloodstream. But even more disturbing to the nurse was the charting of his fluid intake and output and fever, which showed that since Thursday Walter Forsyth's urine output had been declining while his temperature had slowly been rising. Taken together, the evidence left her with little doubt that Forsyth was "going septic" and was already in acute renal failure.

"I'm sick, Striker, sicker now than when I came here," the immense man said as the nurse worked over him. "I told you and I told my son I thought they were doing the wrong things for me here and I know I was right." He sighed wearily, turning his head so the nurse could not see his face. He was silent for a moment before he mumbled almost inaudibly, "I don't want to die, Striker. Not here. I want to go home."

Off guard, the head nurse caught her breath as Forsyth shifted

184

his gaze toward and scrutinized her face, lifting a heavy hand as if to take hold of hers as an expression of incredulity grew in his face. It was a look the head nurse was to carry from the room and recall often after that difficult day had ended. It made her feel, obscurely, as if she were a child standing on a beach watching helplessly as an exhausted swimmer was hauled down by the undertow.

Chapter 31

After Walter Forsyth had died Friday evening, Margaret Striker, assembling his belongings in 324, found a roll of Columbian currency several inches thick and a book of travelers checks, half used, in the amount of $1,750, stuffed in one of his socks. She also discovered, stapled to the tongue of a white patent leather shoe, a waybill indicating that only ten days prior to his admission to the hospital Forsyth had himself shipped several suitcases marked "hold for pick up" from Cartagena to Miami by air freight.

These oddments from the past, hinting at the possibility of intrigue and suggesting that Forsyth had lived among people with deals in their eyes and money in their pockets, believing the "action" had to go on for him, made the head nurse aware of how little anyone on 3H had known of the man and how much had been missing from the brief lesson Dr. Newman had drawn from the drama that had unfolded in 324 that afternoon. For as Margaret Striker had listened to the chief resident's bloodless exegesis of "the facts" of Forsyth's case, she found it rather like hearing someone summarize *King Lear* in medical terms. Missing from Newman's reconstruction of what had happened was the madness, the passion, and the mystery of a journey that had taken Forsyth from lucidity to delirium on his way down to death.

Death had not come stealthily for Walter Forsyth. From the first electrocardiograph that had been done with Margaret Striker's assistance by Dr. Fischer at seven that morning until the last, at three-ten that afternoon, its approach had been tracked with an almost mathematical precision even at the end, when it had come with a ferocious speed.

But governed by the lockstep of routine which was necessary to keep control on 3H, the doctors during the day failed to anticipate the erratic and unexpected pace of events in 324. And though Margaret Striker could not argue with any single decision either Dr. Grossman or Dr. Richards made on Friday, she had sensed, as she watched over Forsyth, that their responses to his deteriorating state were too measured and mechanical to meet the emergency and that just as Newman was later to miss the essential of what had happened to him, both doctors throughout the day on Friday allowed themselves to be so distracted by lab reports and the like that they consistently failed to move rapidly enough to counter the combined effects of sepsis and renal failure that were killing Forsyth.

Forsyth had been increasingly querulous as the hours had ticked by and a morning that began with him demanding to see "the best specialists" and to be moved from 3H to the "private pavilions" ended with him shouting at every doctor and nurse who approached him. Yet despite considerable evidence that his kidney failure was worsening Grossman and Richards had continued to rely on glucose and insulin to try to control Forsyth's elevated serum potassium levels until well past nine o'clock, after they had received the report on the blood sample Mark Eaglesbury had drawn at seven. When it confirmed that Forsyth's serum potassium level two hours before had been a threatening 6.7, Dr. Grossman had given Margaret Striker a stat order for oral kayexelate to counter his "hyperkalemia." But Forsyth's general condition had deteriorated further by then and shortly after ten o'clock—when his fever had reached 101—he had begun vomiting. Uncertain afterward of just how much of the resinous kayexelate Forsyth had retained and how much he had lost, the doctors had rushed a second blood sample off for analysis but in the midmorning confusions in the lab this was evidently misplaced and no report on it was returned to 3H until nearly one o'clock. By then, critical time had been lost. Now in renal shutdown, Walter Forsyth drifted toward delirium and grew increasingly lethargic, and as his ability to concentrate weakened, he had begun to wander the heaths of memory, shouting for lost friends and foes, an enraged and confused old man on his way toward death.

It was at this point that the chief resident had begun to insist that the only way to deal with Forsyth's kidney failure was to perform an emergency peritoneal dialysis to clear his bloodstream of the toxins that were destroying his mind and body. But even as Margaret Striker and Dr. Richards were setting up for the cumbersome procedure, Forsyth had gone into ventricular tachycardia, and shortly afterward Steve Newman odered that a code 700 be called.

As nine doctors and nurses rushed into 324 to crowd shouting at each other around Forsyth's bed, he had become little more than a summary of the last frightening series of numbers that had been returned from the lab and of the long irregular message being printed out by the electrocardiograph. The scene had become nightmarish as they sought frantically to goad his heart into continuing to beat with another machine that sent bolts of electricity into his quivering heart that caused his body to leap and thrash on the bed like a beached fish dying. And when it was over, no one really knew at what point Walter Forsyth had actually died, for the moment had gone by unnoticed, as the doctors and nurses had focused on their equipment and on blood pressure readings, the electrocardiograph, the mechanical maintenance of respiration, and the voltage of the precordial shock, in their frenzy to deny his impending death.

Chapter 32

The head nurse was able to put the scene in 324 out of her mind on Saturday and Sunday. Both were perfect late September days, the sky cobalt, the air like cider, and she spent them happily with

Eliot Cantor as the two confirmed a mutual attraction that was to bind them in a lasting love affair. But when she returned reluctantly to 3H Monday, Margaret Striker knew that Walter Forsyth's death had left its mark on her. Apprehensive about the week of transition ahead, during which Dr. Newman and his interns would be replaced by six strangers and her own staff reduced by Mary Obakwanga's resignation to half what it should be, Margaret Striker found as she made her way through the unit that she was more acutely aware than ever of how much at risk were many of the lives in her charge and how overdrawn already were the floor's resources. Spilling onto 3H, the clear, flat light of September seemed to accentuate its functional sterility, giving a surreal aspect to the place. As she pushed herself through her rounds, it seemed to the head nurse that she glimpsed too often the same fugitive, pleading look she had seen in Walter Forsyth's eyes. It was a look, she realized, that she had seen too many times before and would see too many times again in the faces of other patients —a wordless plea for a miracle that was seldom forthcoming—and Margaret Striker sometimes did not know how to respond to it. More and more of late she found herself wanting to turn away, thinking, "That's somebody else's job—the bedside nurse's job. My job is to keep the ward running smoothly, to try to keep up standards." For she knew that as head nurse she had neither the time nor the energy to become deeply involved with many patients. Yet though she sometimes wished she might be blind, Margaret Striker could not escape the entreaty she saw in the faces of her patients and their families. It was there in Harold Blumenthal's glance when he told her almost shamefacedly on Monday that the doctors had not yet been able to control his bleeding and in the twisted little smile with which Tanya Olsen greeted her each time she entered 316. But while Margaret Striker could give Harold Blumenthal reassurances he found believable, she found as the week wore on that she had no easy answer for the fear that began to flicker first in Tanya Olsen's pale eyes and later in the eyes of her daughter, Caroline, like a silent cry for rescue.

Tanya Olsen was in perilous straits. The deleterious side-effects of her acute form of leukemia and the powerful therapy she had been receiving had both taken their toll of her visibly since her admission to the ward and she seemed to Margaret Striker to have aged by years in a few days. Her chestnut hair, now showing gray at the roots, had become thin and lackluster, and her skin, parched by a continuous fever and marred by small splotches of bruise indicating superficial hemorrhaging, had about it the desiccated fragility of an autumn leaf. For though the poisons had achieved the doctors' immediate goals spectacularly, plummeting her white count from a crisis level of seventy thousand to three thousand in a few days and eradicating cancerous "blast" cells from her bloodstream, the effects of her disease, already well advanced when she had been admitted to 3H, coupled with those of the powerful cytotoxics which had depressed her body's ability to manufacture its own blood supply, by week's end had left her wholly dependent on transfusions to stay alive and so weakened that she had only the frailest of defenses against infection and hemorrhage. And by Monday these defenses had begun to crumble. Tanya Olsen's ulcerated mouth had begun to bleed, she had hemorrhaged slightly into one of her eyes, and the insidious little fever that had burned steadily since she had come to the floor had begun to climb upward, unchecked by antibiotics. But what worried Margaret Striker as much as these threatening indications of the possible onset of a septic crisis due to a secondary fungal infection that antibiotics could not touch was Tanya Olsen's emotional state. Passive from the moment she had arrived on 3H, she had shown neither rage nor grief as she had grown weaker, but instead had seemed almost daily to withdraw further into a province of dream and memory beyond the reach of the professionals who sought to scold and cajole her into rallying to her own defense. Yet when fear sometimes stiffened Tanya Olsen's crooked smile into a rictus, Margaret Striker's stock assurances that "the doctors were well pleased with your response," were useless. The destructive effects of her disease and its treatment, the loss of her hair, the intermittent bone pain, the ulcers in her mouth and bruises on her body were undeniable and as time passed, Margaret Striker, who from the moment she had lain eyes on Tanya Olsen had recognized a peculiar empathy with the slight woman, understood that what she wanted most was acceptance of the truth that she might be dying, and, with it, acceptance of her loneliness and fear as she sought a way to comprehend what was happening to her.

The head nurse had realized this on the previous Friday when she had stopped in 316 to see Mrs. Olsen shortly after Dr. Dorothy Blackmur and her team had made rounds on 3H. Instead of mentioning the hematologists's visit, Mrs. Olsen had begun talking about a television show, though Margaret Striker knew that only moments before Dr. Blackmur had told her that she was entering the most hazardous and uncertain phase of her treatment. Until the bone marrow that had been wiped away by the poisons began to regenerate, not only would she be in acute danger, but no one would know whether she had won a remission from leukemia or whether she would need to submit to another high-risk course of chemotherapy.

"Do you like Barbara Walters?" Tanya Olsen had asked the surprised nurse in a dull tone. "Do you think she's a clever woman?"

"I know very little about her," Margaret Striker had replied, ascribing Tanya Olsen's question to an attempt to deny the importance of what she had just learned by covering it up with small talk. "I'm usually on my way to work when she comes on—or asleep. . . . But why do you ask?"

"Because this morning they were talking about sex on the *Today Show*," had been the unexpected reply. "They were discussing the new morality and sexual freedom and it made me wonder what I'd missed."

Seeing the grave look in Tanya Olsen's face, Margaret Striker had not smiled but had asked gently what she meant. "I mean," Tanya Olsen had answered in a slow, considered voice, "that there seem to be so many things in life I have not experienced—feelings I have missed—that I wonder now if I wasn't too timid of living, if

I didn't cheat myself. . . . But you can't know what will happen to you," she had said quickly. "You go from day to day, that's all. And I had my daughter to raise so I guess I was more careful about keeping the rules." She had continued then, describing to the nurse her brief marriage, her divorce, the years afterward during which she had supported herself and her daughter, Caroline, and finally about the years alone. "When Caroline grew up and married I gave up the apartment we had had. It didn't make sense anymore. I kept my things in three places after that—I had a closet of my own at my daughter's house in New Jersey, one at a friend's apartment in Brooklyn, and then, of course, I had a room of my own near my work. . . . It never seemed temporary before now, but it was, wasn't it?" She had been silent for a moment, her eyes thoughtful. "I missed a lot," she had added, "so I didn't want Caroline to miss anything. I didn't want to move into her house when she asked because I thought it would interrupt her life. She wanted me, though, I know that. So now I must tell her honestly about this thing that is happening to me. And I will. But I want you to explain it to her for me, Margaret," she had said then, reaching for the head nurse's hand and holding it in a gentle grasp. "Not the doctors. You. All Right?"

On Monday, sicker and weaker, in the aftermath of her completed course of chemotherapy, Tanya Olsen had circled closer to her fears when she had recalled for Margaret Striker fragments from her childhood on the farm in Wisconsin as if she sought analogues from the past to guide her in the uncertain present. "My mamma used to tell me," she had mused while the nurse had busied herself hanging up a transfusion pack of red blood cells and normal saline at her bedside, "that the pumpkins weren't ready until the seeds were. She had a way of seeing life in a circle—of seeing birth planted in death and death as a natural harvest." She had given the nurse a lopsided grin at this and then continued, "When my momma died she died at home. My poppa was with her. I remember later, though, when she was in her coffin he took me by the hand and he led me up to kneel beside her and say a prayer. 'There she is,' he said—and he was crying—'the most beautiful woman in the world.' I looked at her. I saw her there—my momma, kinda plain, kinda plump, just my mamma in that coffin and I didn't know what he really meant until a long time later. He loved her, you see. He loved her very much, just like they were still young, right to the end. . . ."

But as her fever climbed upward she burrowed more deeply into herself, as if seeking refuge, barely emerging from her drug-gentled dreams and conscious reveries to speak to the head nurse when she stopped at her bedside.

"Sick," she said on Tuesday as Margaret Striker had taken her vital signs and found her temperature up to 101.3. "Too sick to care. I empty closets in my dreams. I dreamt I lost all my teeth. I saw my mother in her garden. I wake to find people sticking me with needles. Can't they stop? Does it matter so much any more?"

"Bells," she said dreamily that afternoon as the head nurse gently cleansed her ulcerated mouth. "Bells and birds. Please call my daughter. I need her now. And please, no more pain. Let me go."

"Caroline has been here all day," Margaret Striker replied quietly. "She's just outside the door now."

"My mother is dying, isn't she?" said Caroline Matthews, the big woman who was Tanya Olsen's daughter. "She gave up her whole life to me and now she's dying. Oh my God . . ."

Margaret Striker took her by the hand and led her down the corridor to the lounge. "We are fighting for her," she said simply. "Did you talk with Dr. Blackmur after I spoke to you on Friday? Because all that I told you remains true. Ask Dr. Eaglesbury or Dr. Newman. They will tell you your mother still has a chance, a good one."

But on Wednesday, when Margaret Striker came on duty, Tanya Olsen was worse. "Lousy night," Mark Eaglesbury said dourly. "Olsen's now at 102.3 and she had some small convulsions at about three. I don't know . . ."

"Mrs. Olsen's very sick," Marie Velasquez reported, returning to the nursing station at eight-thirty after checking vital signs on A

192

side. "Her pulse rate is up, though the blood pressure is only ninety-five over sixty-five, and the temperature is 103 now."

"Nothing in the smear yesterday, was there, Mark?" Dr. Newman asked after making rounds. "The picture in 316 is dim."

"No blasts," Mark Eaglesbury responded, leaning tiredly on the desk at the nursing station after twenty-eight hours on duty. "But her white count is only six hundred and the question is whether she's leukopenic because she's hypocellular or is the marrow just filling up with blasts again. . . . They're doing another aspiration today."

The fever climbed to 103.2, where it held. Mrs. Olson's daughter paced the hallways or sat stiffly silent at her mother's bedside by the hour.

"The daughter's in trouble," Margaret Striker told the chief resident. "If anything goes wrong she may become hysterical. She wants to know what her mother's chances really are and I don't know what to say."

"Well," the usually sassy chief resident said quietly, doodling on a scrap of paper, "infectious diseases didn't culture up a thing that the Keflin shouldn't have knocked off—bacteria from the mouth ulcers and the like. And without leukocytes we can't locate any abscesses internally . . . yet the fever goes up and holds in the 102–103 range. So it might be fungal, but it might also be meningeal—beyond the blood brain barrier. And it might be intracranial. We did a spinal tap, which was slightly cloudy. We're waiting on that report now."

"Pain," Tanya Olsen cried out, tears streaming down her cheeks. "All pain. Too much pain. They came last night and stuck needles in my spine. I can't go on. Needles and needles. Digging for veins . . . oh, God, I hurt. . . ." Her arms were black and blue, her mouth bloody. She could barely hold up her head as Margaret Striker cleansed her mouth. "I dreamed of my mother again," she said in a voice quiet with resignation. "She prayed beside me and I felt peaceful then . . . and only pain now. . . ."

"Your daughter was here, Mrs. Olsen," Margaret Striker said firmly. "She stayed at your side until very late, I'm told."

"Tell her not to grieve for me if I go," Tanya Olsen answered softly. "Don't anyone grieve."

On Thursday morning Dr. Newman called for a consultation on Tanya Olsen with the hematologists. "Flatl stops 'em dead," said the tall young man with a neatly clipped mustache who arrived from Dr. Blackmur's section. "Only way to get at disseminated fungal infections is flatl. And since the spinal smear shows no reason to suspect meningeal infection—must be fungus. Now, from our side, she could still go either way. Yesterday's marrow aspiration was still hypocellular. She was on a rugged protocol. So the question remains, when will she start making blood—and what will it be? Your job, meantime, is to hang on to her. She's consuming everything she gets every other day in bloods . . . and the fever goes up. Get it down, that's all. Put her on a thermal mattress."

"I'm so cold," Tanya Olsen pleaded, her teeth chattering audibly. "Can't I have extra blankets? Why am I so cold? Margaret, Margaret—I'm so cold and sad, Margaret. Where is my daughter?"

"I sent her for coffee. She'll be back soon. And you're cold because we're making you cold with a thermal mattress to keep your fever down. . . . Please take this now, Tanya—it's Tylenol."

Later that morning the chief resident put Tanya Olsen on the DSL, the dangerously sick list. "We aren't controlling the fever," Dr. Newman acknowledged unhappily, "and the morning counts are still depressed, indicating that she'll need blood again today and she's consuming at a terrific rate. If she needs more blood or platelets than we can get for her over the weekend—well . . ." He drummed his fingers nervously, chewing on his lip. "At present, though, what concerns me is her heart. There have been episodes of tachycardia—atrial tachycardia—but extended enough to be worrisome."

"Is it the Daunomycin?" Dr. Eaglesbury asked bleakly. "I was worried about it's cardiotoxic qualities. . . ."

"That, the fever, the low blood pressure, the anemia, you name it. The heart's not particularly serious with everything else she's got going on, but, Striker, I want it taken by the nurses as a warning signal. I want to hear about any new episodes because if the ventricular rate goes way up, we may have to cardiovert her one of these times."

"Will you tell Mrs. Matthews how things stand, Steve?" Margaret Striker asked. "She's got that wired-up look—you know, her jaws are clenched as tight as her fists lately, and if anything blows she could come apart on us."

"You mean like the guy who came after me when his wife died in July and then tried to fracture his own skull on the wall? Well, I'll speak to her, Margaret—but what's to say? How do you explain anything you haven't got answers for except by saying 'maybe'?" He shrugged, pulled on his mustache, then grinned. "Hey, by the way—you remember what a success the movie *Love Story* was a few years back?"

"Yeah?" the intern and the head nurse responded in chorus.

"Well—they're bringing out a sequel—Ali McGraw returns in 'A *Blast from the Past*.'"

On Friday at noon, moments after Caroline Matthews had arrived at her mother's bedside, Tanya Olsen stopped breathing. The daughter bolted from the room screaming for a doctor and a priest. Newman, his two assistant residents, and five interns were not at the moment on the floor. Closeted in a conference room, the doctors were having a party to celebrate their last day on 3H. Reacting to the emergency, Margaret Striker had slammed down the intercom buttons, paged the chief resident and Mark Eaglesbury, and then dashed for 316. A cursory examination told her that though Tanya Olsen was not breathing there was still a rapid, erratic, and weak pulse. "Tachycardia," she shouted to Ellen King, who appeared in the doorway a moment later. "Probably atrial fib or flutter. Get an ambu, the ECG, and a crash cart in here and where the hell is Newman? He may have to cardiovert if she's hypotensive."

As the head nurse worked over Tanya Olsen she began to breathe again in low, slow, shuddering sighs but despite the nurse's attempt to correct her accelerated pulse rate by massaging the carotid sinuses, Tanya Olsen's heart continued to beat wildly.

"What in Christ's name is going on here?" Mark Eaglesbury snapped, coming into the room to find the head nurse bent over the unconscious Mrs. Olsen. "Why wasn't I paged?"

"'Scuse me, Doctor," said Ellen King, careening into the room, pushing the ECG machine as Marie Velasquez came up behind her with the crash cart and placed it in readiness outside 316. "Do you still need a respiratory assist, Margaret?" Ellen King asked, gesticulating with the small football-shaped pump used in emergencies to ventilate patients who were not breathing on their own.

"A cannula maybe, Doctor?" Margaret Striker responded, turning to Mark Eaglesbury. "No assist, Ellen—she's okay on her own but you will want oxygen, Doctor, won't you? When I got in here she was apneic—in syncope. I think she's in atrial fib—at any rate it's a tachycardia and she is presently hypotensive at ninety over sixty. . . ."

"Okay on the oxygen," Mark Eaglesbury growled, bending over Tanya Olsen to search for signs of hemorrhage. "What else?"

"Well, I tried vagal stimulation—the left carotid—but the heart didn't correct. Pulse rate now in 150. And you *were* paged, Doctor. Twice. You'll want an ECG, won't you?" she asked, reaching into the drawer of the electrocardiograph machine for electrode paste.

"What's going on here?" Newman asked, striding into the room.

"Miss Striker found Mrs. Olsen apneic," the intern answered, "and unconscious. . . . She's in tachycardia still."

"What's the rate, Striker?" the chief resident demanded.

"Then in excess of 150—now 160 and she's increasingly hypotensive. She's dropped from 90 over 60 to 88 over 54—the pulse is still weak, though she's breathing again. . . ."

Newman lifted Tanya Olsen's eyelids to check the pupils and then let his learned fingers play over her neck, flexing it. "No stiffness," he reported.

"No focal signs. Lemme get the ECG going," he snapped as Margaret Striker began affixing the leads in a circle around Tanya Olsen's heart.

"Yeah," Newman said, bouncing on the balls of his feet as the first ECG strip was printed out. "She's in atrial fib, all right, now about 150," he added, tearing off a strip on the first lead and re-counting the rate. "Where's the BP?" he asked.

"Eighty-four over fifty," the head nurse responded, "but it's holding there."

"Let's go to the second lead," Newman ordered crisply.

The serial ECG they ran took several minutes, and as Margaret Striker worked in silence, setting and resetting the leads in a se-quence of twelve combinations to circle Tanya Olsen's heart so that the sensitive stylus picking up its electrical currents, amplified three thousand times, would reflect a complete record of her faulty heart action, she became conscious not only of the hum and scratch of the ECG but of other sounds filtering into 316 from the corridor of 3H. She heard the perpetual static of the public address system garbling a page for a doctor, the voice of her unit clerk complaining "that's not in my job description," a telephone ring-ing shrilly, and beneath it all an unfamiliar moaning sound which she realized at last was coming from Caroline Matthews. The head nurse could see the big woman through the partially opened cur-tains of Tanya Olsen's cubicle. She was standing alone against the wall opposite 316, clutching her large white purse to her breast like someone holding a child. She was rocking slowly back and forth, crooning strangely.

"Well," Dr. Newman said at length, "Mrs. Olsen's just con-verted on her own to a normal sinus rhythm—thank God. She ought to be regaining consciousness as her blood pressure moves up—but let's get her some blood now, Mark, and, Striker, I want you to post a close watch on her vital signs from here on. There's cardiac irritability there for sure—probably the Daunomycin—and one thing this poor lady doesn't need is any more trouble than she's already got. . . ."

Chapter 33

Though Tanya Olsen regained consciousness by the time the priest came to administer the sacrament of the sick, her grip on life seemed to Margaret Striker to have weakened appreciably and for the rest of the day Friday she took little notice of the comings and goings in her room. Instead, dozing intermittently, she seemed to float just under the surface of awareness and though there was sometimes a flicker of interest in her eyes when the head nurse bent over her or a new visitor arrived to take up the vigil in 316, she seemed to have little interest in the continuing struggle for her life or to be conscious of the growing tension among the friends and family gathered at her bedside.

They had come by ones and twos after the morning's crisis to join Caroline Matthews, who had remained, still as a statue, praying at her mother's bedside after the priest's visit, and each time the head nurse returned to check Tanya Olsen's vital signs she found someone new in the room.

The first to arrive, at one-thirty, had been two women. They had stopped just inside the doorway to 316 and stood fumbling nervously with their hands when they had recognized the frail creature in the bed as Tanya Olsen, and had not moved further into the room even after Caroline Matthews greeted them.

Mrs. Matthews' husband had come next; he took his grieving wife's hand and she raised her eyes to his and shook her head. At about three o'clock, while Margaret Striker had been busy hanging a transfusion of whole blood for Mrs. Olsen, her brother had arrived. A small man, he had his sister's sea-pale eyes. The daughter had cried in his arms, rocking herself as before, letting her grief have voice again. The head nurse had brought her coffee from the staff kitchen then and Caroline Matthews, addressing Margaret Striker but speaking to everyone assembled in the room, had said,

"I wanted to take her home. She asked me to. I didn't want her to die here."

As her shift ended at three-thirty Margaret Striker wrote out a pass for Mrs. Matthews, her husband, and her uncle. "If you need to you can stay on after visiting hours tonight," she told Mr. Matthews, "but Mrs. Olsen has not changed at all since this morning and with the transfusions she's received, we don't anticipate any major crisis. Perhaps it would be wiser if you found some place near the hospital to spend the night and took your wife out for a quiet dinner somewhere nearby," she added. "If there's any change in Mrs. Olsen's condition for the worse, you could be called."

On Saturday, amid the confusion created by the changeover of the medical staff, the vigil in 316 continued. "We're keeping Mrs. Olsen on the DSL. It's still very iffy in there today," Dr. Newman told Margaret Striker that morning. "But I've got some good news for you too besides the fact that you won't have to put up with me after today," Newman continued. "Mr. Blumenthal got a gain last night—a good one. The cytotoxics have evidently helped control his antibody response to the AHF and he'll probably be able to go home next week. Now if only you can hang on to Olsen after I'm gone . . ."

At eleven-thirty the new intern who was taking over from Mark Eaglesbury appeared at the nursing station. A slight young man with a sweeping mustache and thinning hair, Dr. Ambler was excited. "That leuk—" he told the head nurse, "that leuk in 316? I just called the lab on her bloods from this morning and she's making! The daughter's crying her head off. It's some scene." He was beaming broadly.

"Her fever's down to 101.2," Mark Eaglesbury confirmed shortly afterward with pleasure. "And her white count went up from six hundred to nine hundred since yesterday. Even the hematocrit's a little better, and though she's obviously not out of the woods with that low a white count, she *is* making blood on her own again."

On Sunday the reports on Tanya Olsen's blood counts were still encouraging. Though still severely depressed, her white count had risen to eleven hundred. When Margaret Striker, who was working through the weekend to help with the transition as Dr. Newman handed over to the new chief resident, Dr. Frobischer, stopped on her rounds to visit in 316, Tanya Olsen had smiled and raised a feeble hand in greeting. "I love this girl," she said softly to her daughter, who returned to her mother's side at ten that morning directly from church. "I think Miss Striker willed me to live, even when I wasn't sure I wanted to. . . ."

By Tuesday Tanya Olsen was strong enough to sit up in bed and her obvious gain in strength was matched on the morning's blood report. Her white count had climbed to twenty-two hundred—her hematocrit had reached thirty-three. The hematologists, encouraged, scheduled a marrow aspiration for the next day to check the quality of her response to therapy.

On Wednesday morning, though her steps were faltering, Tanya Olsen walked on Margaret Striker's arm to the doorway of 316. "I can see down the hall," she said, leaning her head out. "I can see the way out now. I never thought I'd see it again." Beaming, she patted the head nurse's arm. "Whatever they find, I've had my miracle. I won't ask for more," she said.

Three days later Tanya Olsen, at her own request, was signed out of the hospital by her daughter. The new chief resident, infuriated by her decision, listed her discharge as "against medical advice" because Mrs. Olsen had refused to submit to a second marrow aspiration after the one performed on Wednesday had been returned with a report that indicated she might be in remission from leukemia.

But Margaret Striker, who helped her prepare to depart that morning, could only feign joy at the leave-taking, for though she understood that because Mrs. Olsen had come so close to death, she could not bear to have hope taken from her again, the head nurse also knew that if her remission were only partial the slightest infection might easily kill her. Yet she did not try to dissuade Tanya Olsen from her decision, though the new chief resident pressed her to do so, because she realized that even if the cancer still lurked in her bone marrow, Mrs. Olsen did not believe she could withstand another course of poisons. Saying goodbye to her, Margaret Striker felt a bleak sense of incompleteness as she looked down on the small woman whose hair, now white at the roots, stood out in a halo around her face and whose flesh seemed to lie like parchment over her bones, for despite what she had shared with Tanya Olsen in her struggle for life, the head nurse knew she would never see her again and never know how or when her story ended.